Herbal Medicine: Back to the Future

(Volume 4)

Infectious Diseases

Edited by

Ferid Murad (*Nobel Laureate*)
Palo Alto Veterans Hospital California
USA

Atta-ur-Rahman *FRS*
Honorary Life Fellow
Kings College
University of Cambridge
UK

Ka Bian
George Washington University
School of Medicine
Washington
USA

Herbal Medicine: Back to the Future

Volume # 4

Infectious Diseases

Editors: Ferid Murad, Prof. Atta-ur-Rahman, Ka Bian

ISSN (Online): 2542-999X

ISSN (Print): 2542-9981

ISBN (Online): 978-981-14-5871-2

ISBN (Print): 978-981-14-5869-9

ISBN (Paperback): 978-981-14-5870-5

Bentham Science Publishers Pte. Ltd.
80 Robinson Road #02-00
Singapore 068898
Singapore
Email: subscriptions@benthamscience.net

BENTHAM
SCIENCE

CONTENTS

PREFACE

Herbal Medicine: Back to the Future presents expert reviews on the applications of herbal medicines (including Ayurveda, Chinese traditional medicines and alternative therapies). This volume demonstrates the use of sophisticated methods to explore traditional medicine, while providing readers a glimpse into the future of herbal medicine.

The book is a valuable resource for pharmaceutical scientists and postgraduate students seeking updated and critically important information relating to natural product chemistry and pharmacology. The chapters are written by authorities in the field. Chapter 1 reviews the antimicrobial spectrum of allicin (garlic) and carvacrol (oregano) and documents the methods that have currently been used to stabilize or generate the semi-synthetic forms of these compounds. Chapter 2 summarizes the application of polyphenol against infectious diseases caused by bacteria and viruses as pathogens. Chapter 3 describes the experiences of Russians in treating infectious diseases with botanicals—from their earliest recorded history down to the present. Chapter 4 discusses the phytochemical constituents of Azadirachta indica ("neem") with respect to their antimicrobial activity along with possible underlying mechanisms and pathways. Chapter 5 focuses on the role of the novel carriers in the development and revival of herbal medicine.

We hope that the readers involved in the study of infectious diseases will find these reviews valuable and thought provoking so that they may trigger further research on herbal medicines and alternative therapies.

We are grateful for the timely efforts made by the editorial personnel, especially Mr. Mahmood Alam (Director Publications) and Mrs. Salma Sarfaraz (Senior Manager Publications), at Bentham Science Publishers for the publication of this book.

Ferid Murad (Nobel Laureate)
Palo Alto Veterans Hospital
California

Atta-ur-Rahman, *FRS*
University of Cambridge
Cambridge
UK

Ka Bian
George Washington University
School of Medicine
Washington
USA

List of Contributors

Bala Prabhakar	Shobhaben Pratapbhai Patel School of Pharmacy & Technology Management, SVKM's NMIMS, Mumbai, Maharashtra, India
Diana R. Cundell	College of Life Sciences, Thomas Jefferson University, 4201 Henry Avenue, Philadelphia, PA 19128, USA
Inamullah Hakeem Said	Department of life sciences and Chemistry, Jacobs University Bremen, 28759 Bremen, Germany
Mary Schaeffer Conroy	Emeritus Professor, Department of History, University of Colorado, Denver, USA
Monica Joshi	Shobhaben Pratapbhai Patel School of Pharmacy & Technology Management, SVKM's NMIMS, Mumbai, Maharashtra, India
Nikolai Kuhnert	Department of life sciences and Chemistry, Jacobs University Bremen, 28759 Bremen, Germany
Rabab Kamel	Pharmaceutical Technology Department, National Research Centre, El-Bohooth Street, Cairo, Egypt

CHAPTER 1

Improving Anti-Microbial Activity of Allicin and Carvacrol through Stabilized Analogs and Nanotechnology

Diana R. Cundell[1,*]

[1] *College of Life Sciences, Thomas Jefferson University, 4201 Henry Avenue, Philadelphia, PA 19128, USA*

Abstract: Allicin and carvacrol have been appreciated as broad-spectrum antimicrobial agents since the early 20th century and used in both Ayurvedic and traditional Chinese medicines for at least five thousand years. Although research since the 1980s identified several important mechanisms of action for allicin and carvacrol, neither has become part of a classical pharmaceutical regimen. Allicin and carvacrol, like other natural phytochemicals, have been hard to purify and stabilize, which has been a major barrier in their entry into a drug discovery process. During the past two decades, two distinct strategies have changed this position. Bioengineering has allowed allicin and carvacrol to be bound to nanoparticles and immobilized onto coated surfaces or into gels; all these methods maximize the retention of activity coupled with a more targeted release. The fields of synthetic and computational chemistry have long been used to create semi-synthetic and synthetic variants of natural molecules or predict binding strengths of molecules that have improved activity and or bioavailability when compared with the parent compounds. Stabilization using one, or both, of these strategies, has been successful for both allicin (garlic) and carvacrol (oregano). This chapter will review the antimicrobial spectrum of these agents and document the methods that have currently been used to stabilize or generate semi-synthetic forms of each of them. Finally, potential and currently available delivery systems will be explored.

Keywords: Allicin, Carvacrol, Nanoparticles, Natural molecules, Semi-synthetic analogs, Nanotechnology.

GENERAL INTRODUCTION

Even before written records were kept, the man attempted to find interventions for pain and infectious diseases [1]. In searching for ways to relieve symptoms, plants that were available in the local environment and that had been found to be non-toxic and ultimately efficacious were selected by many early cultures [1, 2]. All

* **Corresponding author Diana R. Cundell:** College of Life Sciences, Thomas Jefferson University, 4201 Henry Avenue, Philadelphia, PA 19128, USA; E-mail: Diana.Cundell@jefferson.edu.

Ferid Murad, Atta-ur-Rahman, Ka Bian (Eds.)

this is believed to have begun at least 60,000 years ago with evidence of herbal remedies buried with Neanderthal man [3]. From these trial and error experiences grew the ethnomedicines of Ancient India (Ayurvedic) and China (TCM), which were especially focused on the infections and inflammations common to the region [4]. As the use of ethnomedicines grew, formulations became standardized, providing over 5,000 years of evidence for treatment strategies [1, 4, 5]. Numerous antimicrobial tropical spice plants were used as they were found to prevent food spoilage (*i.e.*, antibacterial) and were used in infection formularies [6]. Chemists began to identify the agents responsible for plant-derived antimicrobials beginning in the early 1900s [7], and it was soon apparent there were numerous secondary metabolites responsible for this activity [8 - 11].

Ironically, although up to one-half of all current pharmaceuticals derive from medicinal plants and the majority relate to their original ethnopharmacological uses [12], few plant-derived antimicrobials have been developed [8]. There are two major reasons for this [13, 14]. Firstly, since the discovery of the soil fungal-derived antibiotic penicillin in 1928, the pharmaceutical industry has focused on natural antibacterial and antifungals from bacteria and fungi rather than plants [13]. Therefore, since the 1950s, few to no antimicrobials have come from any other source, and new antibiotics are typically from chemically modified variants of existing agents [12, 13]. Another barrier to the development of plant-derived antimicrobials was their instability, poor bioavailability, and those extraction methods resulted in variable levels of product composition [14]. Finally, data on herbal medicine efficacy often came from studies that are poorly blinded, contain multiple mixes of plant products, and are not standardized in terms of individual components [15].

With the rapid evolution of resistance to antibacterial and antifungal agents, scientists are now searching for new treatment strategies [16, 17]. Many resistant bacterial or fungal species form biofilms, which are virtually impossible to eradicate even with very high levels of antimicrobial agents [18]. This is an even bigger issue when there are only a few available medications that can be used for those infections. For example, there are only three commonly used medications for the majority of human fungal infections [19 - 22], *i.e.*, Terbinafine (for dermatophyte infections), azole-based medicines like fluconazole and itraconazole for *Candida albicans* and amphotericin B for *Cryptococcus neoformans* [19, 20]. Human pathogens like *C. albicans* and *C. neoformans* are becoming increasingly resistant to fluconazole [18, 20] and amphotericin B [20 - 22]. Plant infections are also usually managed by azole drugs and show an acceleration of resistance [23]. Developing new antifungal and anti-protozoal agents without unwanted side effects has been traditionally more difficult as these eukaryotic microbes share significant structural homology with human cells [17, 24]. The range of existing antiviral [25] medications is also limited.

Creating semi-synthetic or synthetic forms of available medications with improved bioavailability that bypass resistance mechanisms has been relatively successful for antibiotics [26]. Synthetic chemistry allows an analysis of a native molecular structure with the derivation of side chains to improve stability and or bioavailability [27]. This may also be coupled with computational chemistry [27] to predict receptor binding efficacy before the development process begins. Researchers have also returned to look for lead compounds within members of the plant kingdom, and this has proven successful for at least one anti-protozoal [28]. Artemisinin was isolated from wormwood (*Artemisia annua*) in 1973, and since then, stable semi-synthetic analogs of this natural compound are the gold standard in treating malaria [28]. During the past decade, nanotechnology has become the new, effective method to encapsulate and either retain or improve the bioactivity for antibiotics [29] as well as natural antimicrobial herbal compounds [30]. Various formulations have been made, with each providing different advantages of delivery, potency, and bioavailability [29, 30]. Using these same technologies for herbal-derived antimicrobials would increase their tissue bioavailability by decreasing their direct gastrointestinal tract and liver absorption [30].

Are we ready for a new approach to plant antimicrobials? Survey data suggest that between 30 and 80% of people are comfortable using them [8, 15]. Combining traditional knowledge of plant efficacy (ethnomedicine) with computational chemistry and nanotechnology techniques now has the potential to allow us to add these entities to conventional medicines [15]. Of the herbal medicines that have strong antimicrobial activity, allicin (from garlic *Allium sativum* L.) and carvacrol (primarily from oregano *Origanum vulgaris L.*) present themselves as viable candidates. This chapter will discuss the mechanisms of action of each as well as evaluate their current status in the development of stable, bioavailable analogs through both computational chemistry and or nanotechnology techniques. Their chemical structures are depicted in Fig. (**1**).

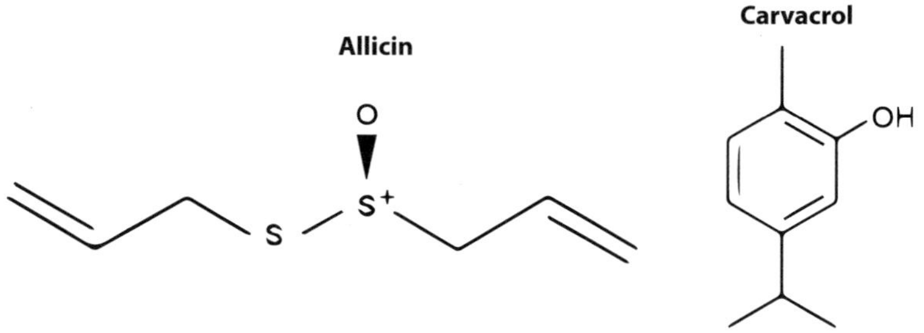

Fig. (1). Chemical structures of allicin and carvacrol.

ALLICIN (FROM GARLIC *ALLIUM SATIVUM* L.)

Introduction

Commercial garlic (*Allium sativum* L.) belongs to a large genus of plants that grow in a wide variety of climates [31] and releases diverse sulfur compounds when crushed or attacked by animals or microbes [32, 33]. Garlic was grown and traded for thousands of years among many early cultures and civilizations for both its nutritional and medicinal properties [34 - 37]. However, not until 1944, with the work of Cavallito and Bailey, were the antibiotic activities of garlic first connected to the organosulfur compound allicin (diallyl-thiosulfinate) [33, 38]. Cavallito and Bailey found allicin was unstable and degraded naturally to produce the less active molecules of diallyl disulfide and trisulfide [33, 38 - 40]. Allicin constitutes at least 70% of the organosulfur molecules in freshly, crushed garlic and can be stabilized for up to 14 days by the addition of alcohol or following drying or freezing [33]. Allicin is now understood to be antibacterial [41], antifungal [42], anti-protozoal [43], antinematodal [43] and antiviral [44], and is non toxic for human cells [32]. Combining allicin with the antifungal agents fluconazole or itraconazole synergistically enhances their *in vitro* killing of *Candida albicans* [45, 46]. Allicin shows additive effects with levofloxacin, cefazolin and ampicillin in the *in vitro* killing of the bacterium *Pseudomonas aeruginosa* [45] and *Mycobacterium tuberculosis*, by chloramphenicol or streptomycin [47]. Garlic cloves contain numerous phytochemicals and so to avoid confusion only studies employing allicin will be discussed in the following sections.

Proposed Antimicrobial Mechanisms of Action for Allicin

Allicin's broad spectrum antimicrobial activities derive from its thiol structure allowing easy penetration of cell membranes and subsequent inactivation of a variety of intracellular [48 - 52] and extracellular [53] targets. Allicin possesses at least seven identificably antimicrobial effects [48 - 78] Fig. (**2**).

Most important among these are biofilm disruption [54 - 57], inhibition of cysteine proteases [48, 49, 52, 58 - 63] disruption of ergosterol transport in fungi [73 - 75] and viral docking and gene synthetic [76 - 78] functions.

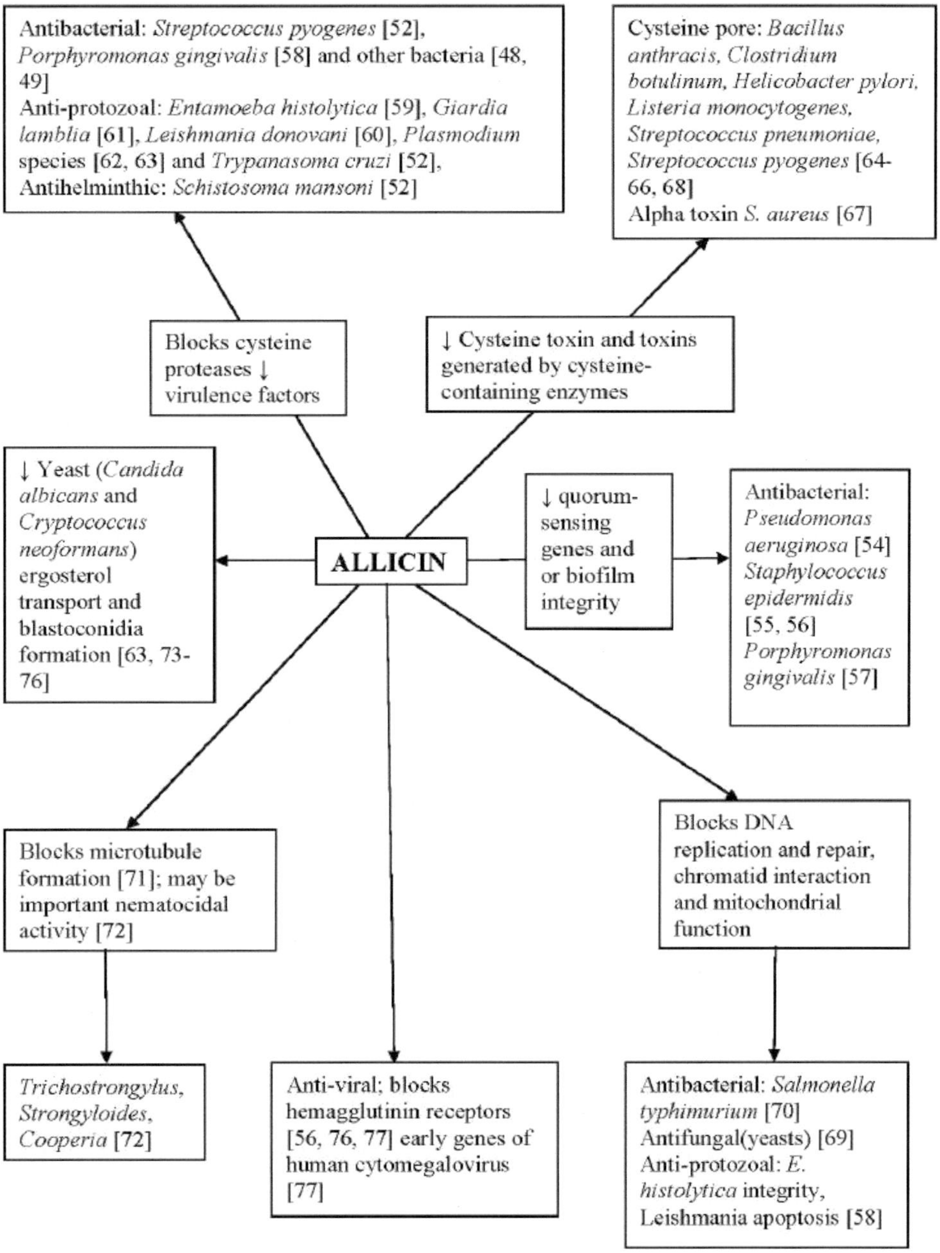

Fig. (2). Possible antimicrobial mechanisms of allicin. Seven potential cellular targets in bacteria, fungi, protozoa, helminths and viruses have been identified for allicin that produce antimicrobial effects (references shown in parentheses).

Biofilm Disrupting Effects of Allicin

At least two mechanisms may be involved [54 - 56]. In bacteria such as *P. aeruginosa* and *Staphylococcus epidermidis* allicin can impair quorum sensing genes, thereby decreasing the ability of the bacteria to form biofilms [41, 54 - 57]. Studies by Zhai *et al.* [56] and Guan *et al.* [57] also suggest a direct bactericidal activity for allicin *i.e.* it can directly penetrate the bacterial biofilm. Zhai *et al.* [56] reported that over a two week period allicin (4 μg/ml) significantly ($p<0.05$) reduced *S. epidermidis* colonization of a femoral implanted screw and washer in New Zealand White rabbits. When vancomycin (20 μg/ml) was co-administered with allicin no biofilm formation was observed [56]. Biofilms increase the antibiotic resistance of bacteria somewhere between 10- and 1,000-fold and therefore any agent able to impair them would be of particular use, therapeutically [54 - 57].

Cysteine-Proteases as Major Targets for Allicin

Microbial cysteine proteases [48, 49], alcohol dehydrogenases [49, 50] and the acetyl-coA system [51] are particularly vulnerable to the effects of allicin and play a major role in its antimicrobial activity. Cysteine proteases in pathogenic microbes are highly conserved [52]. More than three-quarters of all helminth cysteine peptidases and nearly half of all those in protozoan parasites belong to the Clan CA/Family 1 [52]. Allicin's ability to inhibit one such toxin would then extend to many varieties of pathogens. In protozoa, allicin inhibits the cysteine proteases that control production or activation of virulence factors in *Entamoeba histolytica* [58], *Giardia lamblia* [60], *Leishmania donovani* [59] and *Plasmodium* species [61]. Two cysteine protease-sensitive targets associated with protozoal adaptation and invasion have been reported in *Plasmodium* species; the circumsporoite protein (CSP) [79] and falcipain 2 [80]. Studies by Waag [49] reported that allicin was also able to impair *in vitro* activity of the cysteine protease rhodesain from *Trypanasoma brucei* at micromolar levels. Lima *et al.* [81] observed that allicin (5 mg/ml) damaged the outer surface of *Schistosoma mansoni* and caused ulcers to form *in vitro*. Calpain from *S. mansoni* is expressed in the external (tegument) layer of *S. mansoni* [82]. Allicin binding to this surface protein may go some way to explaining the observations of Lima *et al.* [81]. Cysteine proteases are essential in processing hemoglobin for nutrients in bloodborne parasites [83] so allicin could be a useful against many species.

Allicin Targets Bacterial Cysteine-Containing Toxins and Alpha Toxins

Allicin is able to inhibit the highly conserved, cysteine-containing, pore-forming bacterial exotoxins of a further seven bacterial species including the important pathogens *Bacillus anthracis, Clostridium botulinum, Helicobacter pylori,*

Listeria monocytogenes, Streptococcus pneumoniae and *S. pyogenes* [41]. Allicin's binding of their central cysteine residue results in toxin inactivation and elimination of bacterial pathogenesis [64 - 66]. Alpha toxins, which are pore forming but contain no cysteine [84], are also inhibited by allicin. Studies by Leng *et al.* [66] suggest that allicin inhibits the transcription of the *agr* (accessory gene regulator) of *S. aureus* alpha toxin. Agr proteins, require an active cysteine for full functionality [85], so this might provide a second target for allicin. Ranjbar-Omid *et al.* [68], reported that allicin (7 µg/15 ml) was able to inactivate the urease from *Proteus mirabilis*.This, they suggest, is due to allicin targeting the cysteine group present in the urease [68].

Allicin Affects Microtubule Polymerization

Studies of fibroblasts [71] and plant-derived intestinal nematodes [72] have suggested that allicin may affect microtubule polymerization. Allicin and albendazole were not additive effects [72], suggesting they may be targeting similar pathways. Albendazole is a tubule inhibiting agent [86] an effect also reported for allicin [72] and this may explain its nematocidal activities.

Allicin Inhibits Ergosterol Transport in Yeasts

Anti-yeast activities may involve the ability of allicin to prevent the cellular protective response of ergosterol (fungal cholesterol) transport to the internal vacuoles that are central to their survival [63]. Studies by Borjihan *et al.* [63], compared the effects of amphotericin B (AmB) and allicin on *C. albicans* and reported these involved similar effects on the internal vacuoles. Khodavandi *et al.* [74] reported that allicin damaged the *C. albicans* cell surface. These authors also reported allicin affected *C. albicans* blastoconidia germination and hyphal formation [75].

Allicin Binds to Docking Receptors Preventing Viral Entry and Gene Synthesis

Highly conserved, viral hemagluttinin receptors on mammalian cells also contain thiol sulfur groups [76, 78]. These docking receptors are used by many viruses including Epstein Barr Virus (EBV), hepatitis C and human cytomegalovirus (HCMV) to enter host cells [44] and appear to be inactivated by allicin [56]. HCMV attaches to host cells using these types of receptors [44] and allicin could prevent both viral binding and replication using these mechanisms. Feng *et al.* [77] reported that growth of a viral cycle protein mutant of HCMV (IE72) was relatively unaffected by stabilized allicin (Allitridin™), whereas that of a clinical strain (A169) was significantly reduced ($p<0.001$) [77]. Allitridin™ inhibited early phase viral antigen E protein production [77]. If these studies translated to human HCMV infection it would represent a novel and unique way to intervene with these infections, which have no vaccine and are deadly in neonates [34].

Spectrum of Allicin's Antimicrobial Activity

Antibacterial

Recently reviewed by Wagner-Graham [41], allicin possesses broad-spectrum *in vitro* bactericidal activity against the majority of both gram-positive and gram-negative bacteria that have been investigated. Studies comparing allicin's effects with conventional antibiotics have reported differential sensitivity depending on the bacterial strain being investigated [79, 83]. Reiter *et al.* [87] suggested that allicin required significantly lower ($p<0.05$) minimum inhibitory concentrations (MIC) than clindamycin and erythromycin against antibiotic-resistant strains of *Streptococcus pneumoniae*. Some oral pathogens seem to be particularly susceptible to allicin with the periodontal pathogen *Aggregatibacter actinomycetemcomitans* demonstrating an MIC of 4.1 μg/ml, whereas the notoriously resistant *Porphyromonas gingivalis* displayed an MIC of 22.7 μg/ml [82]. Kulik *et al.* [88] recently surveyed strains of *A. actinomycetemcomitans* and *P. gingivalis* and reported an MIC range of between 0.25 and 32 μg/ml to conventional antibiotics. Antibiotic-resistant bacteria killed by allicin include MRSA [89, 90], vancomycin-resistant *Enterococci* (VRE) [91] and *M. tuberculosis* (MDR-TB) [92].

Only nine bacteria show limited responses to the effects of allicin [93 - 96]. Five of these are *Pseudomonas* or formerly ascribed to the *Pseudomonas* genus [93]. Bacteria were originally not believed to cross-transfer resistance to allicin [97] but recent studies with the garlic bulb pathogen *P. fluorescens*, suggest this is not the case [98]. Allicin resistance genes controlled redox functions and Borlinghaus *et al.* [98], hypothesized these had allowed the *P. fluorescens* to colonize garlic.

Allicin-resistant *P. aeruginosa* [99], *C. acidovorans* [100], *S. maltophilia* [101] and *Flavimonas oryzihabitans* [102] are all plant-associated, environmentally-acquired species that could easily perpetrate this gene transfer with the garlic colonizing *P. fluorescens*. *Erwinina* [102] are also plant pathogens that readily exchange genes with *P. fluorescens*. Allicin is able to inhibit not only human and plant bacterial pathogens but also those affecting primarily fish [104 - 106]. Farmed grass carp [105, 106] and rainbow trout [107] administered allicin for between 30 and 60 days significantly ($p<0.05$) reduced their incidence of infection rates and demise from waterborne bacteria, particularly *Aeromonas hydrophilus*. Allicin was also shown in these studies to improve the animals' innate immune system effects [104 - 107] and growth rates [105, 106].

Antifungal

The antifungal activities of allicin were recently reviewed by French-Arthur [42] and, although lesser in number of both studies and spectrum of activity, are notable for the species affected. Six studies investigated the efficacy of allicin against the human pathogenic yeasts *Candida albicans* [42, 74, 75, 93, 108] and *Cryptococcus neoformans* [91, 108, 109]. Allicin was as effective against four other pathogenic *Candida* species [93] and against the dermatophytes *Trichophyton, Epidermiphyton* and *Microsporum (*MIC 3.13-6.26 μg/ml) [96]. MIC values for *A fumigatus* were slightly higher at between 12.5 and 12.5-25 μg/ml [108, 110]. Allicin (5 mg/kg/day) increased the survival of mice infected with *A. fumigatus* [110]. Intravenous treatment with allicin allowed the *A. fumigatus*-infected mice to survive for nearly three weeks and oral treatment for two weeks compared with only a week for untreated animals [110].

Allicin has been investigated in two studies as a plant antifungal and shown efficacy against four fungal species [111, 112]. Curtis *et al.* [111] reported that allicin (280 μg) inhibited the *in vitro* growth of the plant fungi *Alternaria brassisicola, Botrytis cinerea, Magnaporthe grisea,* and *Plectosphaerella cucumerina*. These authors also noted that a 700 μg/ml allicin spray was able to impair the germination of *M. grisea* spores on rice [112]. A second study by Parvu *et al.* [112] found that allicin was able to kill *Fusarium oxysporum* but with a higher MIC (160 μg/ml) than the standard treatment of fluconazole (100 μg/ml).

Anti-protozoal and Anti-helminthic

Allicin has been shown to possess *in vitro* [58, 60, 61, 70, 113, 114] and *in vivo* [61, 62, 95, 115] anti-protozoal activities against four human pathogens. Studies suggest this is primarily mediated through allicin's inactivation of cysteine proteases [59 - 61, 115]. Allicin (10-50 μM) significantly ($p<0.05$) reduced viability of active forms of the protozoa *Entamoeba histolytica* [59, 113], *Giardia duodenalis* [60], *Leishmania infanta* and *L. donovani* [114] and *Plasmodium berghei* [61]. Corral *et al.* [115] observed that allicin (15-120 μM) produced effects after only three hours of *in vitro* incubation and that this resulted in cell cycle arrest of *L. infantum*. Allicin (5 or 8 mg/kg/day) was also reported to be effective in rodent models of leishmaniasis [95, 115] and malaria [61, 62]. In these studies, allicin significantly ($p<0.001$) increased animals' survival from both infections [61, 62, 95, 115]. Combining allicin with AmB (1 mg/kg/day) resulted in a >95% clearance of *L. infantum* from a hamster model of leishmaniasis [115].

Finally, allicin is anti-helminthic [81, 116, 117]. Metwally *et al.* [116] reported elimination of *S. mansoni* liver and intestinal burden after 8 weeks in mice following treatment with allicin (0.5 μM by gavage). Allicin significantly decreased (p<001) hatching of *Meloidogyne incognita* eggs and penetration of the nematode into treated tomato seedlings (25 ppm for 5 minutes) [117].

Anti-viral

Both *in vitro* [77, 118 - 120], *in vivo* animal studies [77, 121, 122] and two human DBRPCT studies [123, 124] have appeared in the literature in support of allicin possessing antiviral activities. Modest changes of between 1 and 2 log differences were reported in the single *in vitro* study for the viral growth of human papillomavirus (HPV), human rhinovirus (HRIV) and herpes simplex virus (HSV) exposed to allicin (25-1,000 μg/ml) [121]. Stability may have been an issue for native allicin as *in vitro* [118] and *in vivo* [77, 118] animal studies of HCMV using Allitridin™ demonstrated efficacy at low levels (7.5 or 25 μg/ml) [77, 118]. Allicin/ Allitridin™ (0.2-5 g/kg/day) decreased viral load and prevented the demise from HCMV and the lethal poultry conditions of infectious bursal disease virus (IBDV) and reticuloendotheliosis (REV) [77, 121, 122].

Human DBRPCT of allicin as an upper respiratory infection antiviral did not identify the viruses involved but did report a produce a significant decrease in symptoms (p<0.001) [123, 124]. Josling [123] found that adults (n = 146) given allicin (180 mg/day/ 12 weeks) exhibited only one-third of the cold symptoms as that of a placebo group. Andrianova *et al.* [124] found a similar decrease in upper respiratory tract symptoms in a study of children (n = 83), using the proprietary Allicor™ (0.3 mg/ day) stabilized form of allicin. Given that rhinoviruses are the most common virus associated with colds (90% of all cases) [125] these studies may reinforce the earlier finding of allicin's *in vitro* activities against the HRIV [119].

Semi-synthetic Allicin Analogs

Five literature studies have reported the creation of analogs of allicin and tested them against bacteria [94, 126 - 128] or fungi [94, 126 - 129]. Each study has provided more clues as to how to improve the bioactivity of allicin against gram-positive bacteria that include increasing chain length [80, 126, 128] and pentyl substitutes [80, 126] (Table **1**). Most promising as broad-spectrum agents of the allicin analogs were those consisting of cycloalkyl and aryl esters of 4-acylamino-4-acylaminobenzenethiofulfoacids [127]. Although no direct stability data was provided for these analogs, cycloalkyl and aryl substitutions are typically more stable than the parent compound [130]. Qi *et al.* [129] report the synthesis of an *S*-ethyl ethanethiosulfinate allicin analog with both superior antifungal activity and stability. With the exception of the study by Small *et al.* [126], the remaining synthetic allicin analogs have all been designed in the past five years and none tested in animal models for antimicrobial activity. These studies do, however, give us an insight into how allicin might be modified for future mainstream use.

Table 1. *In vitro* antimicrobial activity of semi-synthetic analogs of allicin.

Analogs Created	Results	References
Alkyl analogs created using peracids tested using 20 bacteria	Branched alkyl chains ↓ activity (10-1, 200 μM). *n*-penty- -thiosulfinate ↑stable and bactericidal (0.7 to 130 μM).	[126]
Twenty-four aminobenzene sulfur acid analogs tested positive and 6 gram-negative bacteria and 8 fungi	Broad-spectrum antimicrobial activity for cycloalkyl and aryl esters of 4-acylaminobenzenethiofulfoacids. Acyl residues substituted with fluorine were strongly fungicidal. Thiosulfinates were most effective against gram-positive bacteria, less so against gram-negative.	[127]
Nineteen pyridyl disulfide analogs tested against a 10 species panel of bacteria.	Antibacterial activity against staphylococci and enterococci (VRSA and VISA) was maximal using pyridyl disulfide analogs (MIC 1.56 -25 μM). Gram-negative bacteria were insensitive.	[128]
Four variants of allicin tested against 3 gram-negative bacteria, 1 gram-positive bacterium and a yeast	DMTS, DETS, DPTS and DBTS effective against *Saccharomyces cerevisiae.* Allicin, DMTS and DETS) effective against *Pseudomonas syringae* (MIC 16-32 μg/ml). Allicin, DPTS and DBTS effective against *Micrococcus luteus* (MIC 16-32 μg/ml).	[94]
S-ethyl ethanethiosulfinate (ALE) tested against *Penicillium chrysogenum,*	ALE had an IC_{50} against *P. chrysogenum* of 0.92 μg/ml (compared with 38.68 μg/ml for allicin). ALE↓ mycelial production and spore viability. Stability of ALE was ↑ compared with allicin.	[129]

Abbreviations: Dimethyl-thiosulfinate (DMTS), diethyl-thiosulfinate (DETS), dipropyl-thiosulfinate (DPTS) and dibenzyl-thiosulfinate (DBTS)-thiosulfinate, IC_{50} (half maximal inhibitory concentrations), MIC (minimum inhibitory concentration), VISA (vancomycin intermediate *S. aureus*), VRSA (vancomycin-resistant *S. aureus*).

Nanoparticle and Immobilized Allicin Studies

Seven studies have stabilized the antibacterial and antifungal activity of allicin [131 - 137] (Table **2**). Nanoparticle (NP) derivatives were the most popular strategy used with four of the six studies investigating allicin alone [131, 133, 135, 136] or in combination with antibacterial silver [135, 136]. NP allicin was significantly ($p<0.001$) more effective in three of the four studies [131, 135, 136] than native allicin. Allicin and silver were additive in rapidly eliminating murine *S. aureus* skin infections [135, 136]. Antifungal NP [131] and cellulose-complexed [134] forms of allicin have provided an extended, stable release of the thiosulfinate. Nanocomposite woven and non-woven allicin-coupled fabrics displayed *in vitro* antibacterial activity against both *S. aureus* [133, 135] and *E. coli* [135]. Fabrics created using this process could be safely laundered for between 2 [135] and 6 washes [133] without the loss of activity. More recently Soumya *et al.* [138] prepared locust bean gun allicin-coupled NP and demonstrated their lack of toxicity following ingestion by Sprague Dawley rats.

Table 2. ***In vitro*** **antimicrobial activity of nanoparticle and immobilized allicin.**

Study Design	Results	References
PBCA NP containing allicin prepared and investigated for antifungal activity	Dermatophyte MIC 1.46 μg/ml and 2.93 μg/ml for *Candida albicans*. Prolonged release.	[131]
Allicin was complexed with chitosan by freeze drying (yield ~65%)	Good antibacterial activity against gram-positive and gram-negative bacteria.	[132]
Cellulose NP conjugated separately with allicin and lysozyme.	Antibacterial and antifungal effects (MIC 500 μg/ml). Higher than the MIC for allicin (62.5-250 μg/ml) but more stable.	[133]
Allicin-conjugated nanocellulose evaluated using AATCC test method 100–1993	Effective in killing *S. aureus* (>99% killed). Textile could also be safely laundered twice.	[134]
Ag +/- allicin incorporated into NP (10-30 μM) ointment. Ointment spread onto MRSA-infected wounds on murine skin and bacterial numbers counted after 4 days	MIC of allicin and Ag nanoparticles were 2.2 mg/mL and 5.6 mg/ml. Combining resulted in an MIC of 0.4 mg/ml. No bacteria were recovered from murine skin using Ag + allicin.	[135]
Ag alone or with allicin NP introduced on murine *S. aureus* skin infections	Ag NP *S. aureus* MIC 6.25 μg/ml, allicin NP 10.68 μg/ml. Ag+ allicin MIC 1.33 μg/ml.	[136]
Cerium oxide (CeO_2)-allicin nanocomposites in woven and non-woven fabrics tested against *E. coli* and *S. aureus*	CeO_2-allicin fabric bactericidal (>99% killed) *in vitro* after 24 h of bacterial culture. Activity maintained up to 6 washes.	[137]

Abbreviations: Ag (silver), MIC (minimum inhibitory concentration), MRSA (methicillin-resistant *S. aureus*), NP (nanoparticle), PBCA (polybutylcyanoacrylate).

CARVACROL (FROM OREGANO *ORIGANUM VULGARE* L.)

Introduction

Woody plants of the genus *Lamiaceae* tribe Menthae includes important medicinal herbs of the oregano (*Origanum*) family [139]. Oregano, particularly *Origanum vulgare* L., is a native plant that is widespread across temperate and semi-tropical climates [140, 141]. These plants have been used for thousands of years for treating infectious diseases [142 - 144]. Oregano is rich in terpene-containing essential oils (EO) including carvacrol, thymol, γ-terpinene and *p*-cymene [140]. Between 10 and 90% of the EO of *Origanum vulgare* (depending on sub-species and culture conditions) is now understood to be the antimicrobial terpene carvacrol [140] with lesser amounts (~10%) seen in of its thymol isomer [140].

Carvacrol is a monoterpenoid, phenol compound with the formula 2-methyl-5-propan-2-xylphenol [145]. It was first isolated by German chemist Friedrich Carol Voelckel in 1840 from the oil of the unrelated plant caraway seed (*Carum carvi*) [146]. Edward Schweizer gave carvacrol its name in 1842 [147] and by 1918 carvacrol was a recognized prominent component in all *Origanum* species [148]. Since then, carvacrol has been shown to exert potent antifungal [149 - 151] and antiviral RNA- [152 - 154] and DNA-containing virus activities [155]. Carvacrol also possesses antibacterial [149, 156, 157], anti-protozoal [158 - 160] and nematicidal [149, 161] efficacy. The terpene shows synergism with conventional therapies [149, 156], damaging bacterial membranes and improving entry of antibiotics [162 - 164]. Carvacrol is stable to heating [161, 162] and retains activity at room temperature [164] although it remains relatively volatile [165]. Mild heating may even improve its antibacterial activity [162, 163]. Being an organic monoterpenoid, gives natural carvacrol poor bioavailability [166 - 168].

EO derivatives have proven especially appealing especially for organic produce [169] as a safer substitute for antibiotic treatment of livestock [170 - 172]. Oral care and the dental industry may be another direction for carvacrol development [173, 174]. Modifications of natural carvacrol to improve its utility include adding an adjuvant, to increase bioavailability [175], incorporation into nanoparticles [176 - 179] or bonding to surfaces [165]. Many of the reports of stabilized carvacrol have only appeared as published studies within the past three years [177 - 180] with all authors reporting enhanced stability [165, 176 - 180], water solubility [165], shelf life [165] and antimicrobial activity [176 - 180].

Proposed Antimicrobial Mechanisms of Action for Carvacrol

Ultee *et al.* [181] identified that much of the antimicrobial activity of carvacrol was attributable to its free hydroxyl (OH) group and allowed it to act as an active exchanger of protons, weakening the cell membrane by disturbing the phospholipid bilayer. Ben Arfa *et al.* [182] confirmed the requirement of the OH group for activity. Several elegantly constructed studies suggest that natural phenols like carvacrol, thymol and eugenol, are able to easily penetrate and incorporate themselves into phospholipid films as well as binding to γ-aminobutyric acid (GABA) receptors [183 - 185]. Reiner *et al.* [183], using monolayer Langmuir films, confirmed that these phenols were able to expand the monolayer and locate themselves next to the phosphate groups of these molecules. Using phospholipid liposomes this same group further reported that these moieties were fully able to partition into these model membranes [184]. Finally, the more recent studies by Miguel *et al* [185], using a l-2-dipalmitoyl-sn-glyc-ro-3-phosphocholine (DPPC) bilayer, reported carvacrol showed a not dissimilar partitioning spectrum into as the general anesthetic propofol. Miguel *et al* 185] concluded that carvacrol and other phenols *"locate in the region between the polar group (choline molecule), the glycerol and the first atoms of the acyl chains."* This would explain the bacterial membrane disruption seen by other authors [181, 182]. Although not the topic of this chapter, it may also provide another potential use for small phenols; that of modulating the pain-reducing GABA receptor [183 - 185].

Churklam *et al.* [186] observed that carvacrol produced cell membrane degeneration and compromised mitochondrial function in *L. monocytogenes*, resulting in cell lysis [186]. Reduced bacterial intracellular ATP following carvacrol exposure has been reported from *in vitro* studies of *Escherichia coli* and *Listeria monocytogenes* [187, 188]. Gill and Holly [188], found that carvacrol (5-10 mM) depleted intracellular ATP by binding to the bacterial cell membrane ATPase, thereby killing the bacteria. Carvacrol possesses at least six other targets in microbial cells [150, 160, 189 - 200] (Fig. **3**).

Important bacterial targets of carvacrol include impairing flagellar expression [188 - 190] and biofilm formation [173, 189 - 196]. Antifungal activities of carvacrol revolve around preventing biofilm formation [197, 198] and disrupting ergosterol biosynthesis [150, 199, 200]. Carvacrol can deplete the human analog of ergosterol, cholesterol from cell membranes preventing human immunodeficiency virus (HIV) [152] entry. Literature reports show carvacrol kills protozoal oocysts [160] and prevents norovirus [154] and herpes virus [155] replication. Most exciting is the recent report that carvacrol can bind to the major protease (M^{pro}) for severe acute respiratory syndrome coronavirus-2 (SARS-Co--2) COVID-19 preventing its replication [153].

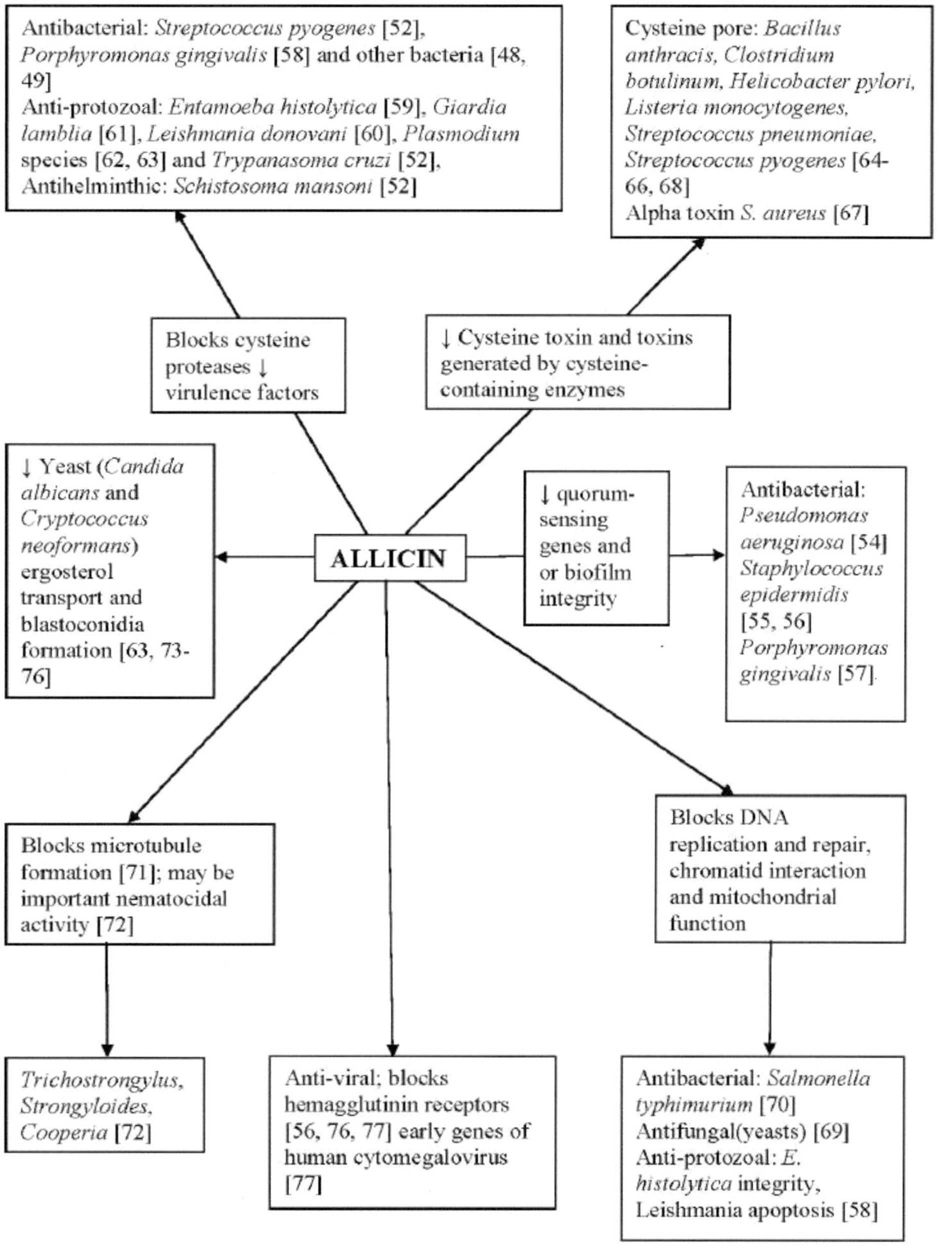

Fig. (3). Possible antimicrobial mechanisms for carvacrol. Seven potential targets in bacteria, fungi, protozoa and viruses have been identified by researchers for curcumin that are responsible for its antimicrobial effects. Abbreviations: OH (hydroxyl).

Biofilm Disrupting Effects of Carvacrol

Carvacrol is able to inhibit the formation of bacterial [189, 190, 192 - 196] and fungal [197, 198] biofilms. Several quorum sensing genes are carvacrol targets [173, 190, 192, 195] Although primarily hydrophobic, carvacrol possesses sufficient amphipathic qualities to allow it to penetrate the polysaccharide outer coatings of mature bacterial biofilms [149]. Literature studies have reported rapid effects, within 5 minutes, of administering sub-lethal doses of carvacrol to *in vitro* biofilms of *C. jejuni* [190], *P. fluorescens* [191], *S. aureus* [193], *S. epidermidis* [193] and *S. typhimurium* [196]. Carvacrol also prevented the *in vitro* formation of *C. albicans* [197], *Cryptococcus neoformans* and *C. laurentii* [198] biofilms.

Aromatic alcohols are believed to regulate fungal quorum sensing activities during environmental stress conditions [201]. Phenols react with alcohols to form O- and C- alkylated products [202] so it is possible that carvacrol could inactivate these aromatics, thereby switching off biofilm initiation. Carvacrol may act on the secondary phase of biofilm formation [197]. Analysis of the pre-formed *C. neoformans* biofilms following exposure to carvacrol or amphotericin B (AmB), revealed they displayed similar surface changes [198]. AmB attaches to ergosterol in the fungal cell membrane and causes pores to form, which through ion egress, result in cell death [203]. Given carvacrol's reported effects on ergosterol [150, 199] it is likely that fungal biofilm dispersal may involve membrane damage.

Oxidative Stress Effects of Carvacrol

Bacteria respond to oxidative stress and reactive oxygen species (ROS) by upregulating their levels of unsaturated fatty acids and shifting their metabolism to a fermentative kind [173, 204, 205]. Exposure to sublethal doses of carvacrol (2.06 mM or 50% MIC) in the presence of a pulsed electric field doubled the levels of unbranched fatty acids in *S. aureus* [204], *E. coli, L. monocytogenes* and *Salmonella enteritidis* [205]. These studies suggest carvacrol prevents stress adaptation in bacteria, resulting in their demise. Using sublethal carvacrol concentrations may favor resistance development in some bacteria [206].

Carvacrol Inhibits Flagellar Gene Expression

Pathogenic bacteria that possess flagella utilize them for migration, targeted adherence to host cell surfaces and biofilm formation [207 - 210]. Wagle *et al.* [190] reported that carvacrol (0.13 mM) significantly downregulated ($p<0.05$) the expression of three *C. jejuni* flagellar genes following 48 hours of exposure. Exposure of *E. coli* [189] and *P. fluorescens* [191] to sublethal doses of carvacrol significantly ($p<0.05$) downregulated the flagellin genes flic and FlgA, respectively.

Carvacrol Decreases Cell Membrane Ergosterol and Cholesterol Levels

Carvacrol (0.005-0.01%) disrupts calcium levels in *S. cerevisiae via* a similar pathway as that initiated during the "calcium stress response" [211]. Analysis of gene transcripts confirmed carvacrol affected the TOR (Target of Rapamycin) pathway, which regulates mobilization of sterols from the endoplasmic reticulum (ER) [212]. Disruption of this pathway would reduce eukaryotic membrane sterol levels [212]. Carvacrol impairs *in vitro* membrane sterol levels in fungi (ergosterol) [149, 199, 201] and human cells (cholesterol) [152]. Chaillot *et al.* [213] suggested compromised ER integrity resulted in the observed sterol and calcium changes in *C. albicans* produced by carvacrol [213].

Carvacrol Affects Viral Particle Replication

Studies by Gilling *et al.* [154] reported that carvacrol (0.5%) murine noroviral capsid proteins, causing the virus to swell and preventing its attachment to RAW 264·7 cells. These data were supported by the findings of Sharif-Rad *et al.* [155] using the DNA-containing herpes simplex virus, HSV-1. Another study on HSV-1 reported carvacrol had no effect on the viral genome, suggesting carvacrol prevented viral entry to host cells [214]. Herpes simplex viruses are known for their genetic diversity [215] and recent studies suggest that HSV-2 may respond differently to carvacrol [216]. Wang *et al.* [216], reported that carvacrol's (2%) ability to decrease HSV-2 infection of Vero and BSC-1 cells involved both viral gene and host cell effects. Another viral major replication protein potentially affected by carvacrol is the main protease (M^{pro}) of severe acute respiratory COVID-19 [153]. Using computational chemistry structural analysis, Kumar *et al.* [153] predicted strong binding of carvacrol to the active pocket of the COVID-19 M^{pro} enzyme. This is an exciting finding as M^{pro} is considered the most vulnerable protein in COVID-19 and would provide an optimal target against the virus [217].

Other Possible Carvacrol Activities

Wang *et al.* [201] reported that carvacrol bound to the minor groove of DNA *via* hydrogen bonds. These authors stated this binding affected the secondary structure of DNA and caused its aggregation [204]. Kortman *et al.* [218] reported carvacrol prevented *S. typhimurium* colonization of human Caco-2 cells by preventing bacterial uptake of iron. Carvacrol (0-0.5 mM) was shown to directly remove iron from transferrin in this study [218].

Spectrum of Carvacrol's Antimicrobial Activity

Antibacterial Activity

Recently reviewed by Marchese *et al.* [219], carvacrol has been reported to possess activity against over twenty common food-borne and human clinical strains of gram-positive and negative bacteria. Also included are the important antibiotic-resistant bacteria MRSA [220, 221], VRE [221] and resistant group A streptococci [156]. Carvacrol inhibits several bacterial toxins including *S. aureus* coagulase and enterotoxin [222], *Clostridium difficile* toxin [223], listeriolysin O from *L. monocytogenes* [224], *Vibrio cholera* toxin [225], enterohemorrhagic *E. coli* (EHEC) toxins [226]. These effects are thought to be mediated through direct downregulation of genes coding for these toxins [223 - 225]. Native carvacrol is much weaker against gram-negative bacteria (MIC 0.01 and 5 mg/ml) than conventional antibiotics [219, 222, 226]. Carvacrol MIC values for gram-positive bacteria range between 0.04 and 256 mg/ml [220], which is comparable with those for conventional antibiotics [227]. A more promising strategy for carvacrol may be to use it to potentiate existing antibiotics [156, 221, 228, 229]. Synergy between carvacrol and erythromycin [156], amikacin [221], tetracycline [228], bacitracin [229] and colistin [229] has been reported. Other studies have reported no synergy with erythromycin [228], so the effects may be species dependent. Cirino *et al.* [228] demonstrated carvacrol inhibited the tetracycline efflux pump, with no effects on efflux pumps for erythromycin or norfloxacin.

Antifungal

Carvacrol has been demonstrated to possess *in vitro* activity against at least seventeen varieties of human pathogenic fungi [150, 197 - 200, 219, 230 - 234] and seven plant pathogens [235 - 239]. *Candida* and *C. albicans* strains have been extensively studied with carvacrol displaying MIC values of between 0.04 and 0.5 µg/ml [219, 231, 232]. Studies by Chami *et al.* [151, 240] reported carvacrol (1,000 µg/ml) was able to eliminate *C. albicans* infection of the mouth and vagina in dexamethasone (0.5 mg/L)-suppressed rats. Aspergillus strains, including *A. niger* and *A. fumigatus* are susceptible to carvacrol (MIC 16-32 µg/ml) [230, 231, 233]. Literature studies have reported dermatophytes are the most sensitive with MIC of 0.04-0.16 µl/ml [230, 231, 234]. These MIC data are compatible with standard antifungals [20, 22], suggesting carvacrol as a good potential lead for new medications. Carvacrol potentiates the effects of conventional antifungal agents [232, 235]. Ahmad *et al.* [232] reported carvacrol decreased the fluconazole efflux from resistant *C. albicans* strains by inhibiting the major genes *CDR1* and *MDR1*. Jesus *et al.* [236] observed a reduction in MIC of between 64 and 96% for four antifungal agents against the plant and human pathogen *Pythium insidiosum*.

Carvacrol or carvacrol-enriched EO has been shown to inhibit seven common fungal plant pathogens [235 - 239]. Low concentrations of carvacrol (1.0-5.0 mM) completely prevented the *in vitro* mycelial growth of *Botryodiplodia theobromae* [237], *Colletotrichum acutatum* [237], *Fusarium* sp [234], *Phytophthera capsici* [236] and *Rhozoctonia solani* [236]. Carvacrol (1.0 mM) irreversibly destroyed cell membrane of the peach rot pathogen *Rhizopus stolonifera* [239]. Fumigation of peach plants (2 µl) and inoculating harvested peaches (0.5 µl/ml) with carvacrol prevented peach rot developing [239].

Anti-protozoal and Anti-helminthic

Only a few studies have appeared in the literature that discuss anti-parasitic effects for carvacrol, but these have all suggested it is a potent agent [158 - 161]. *In vitro* studies of carvacrol (IC_{50} or half maximal inhibitory concentrations<0.4 mg/ml) reported lysis of the resistant oocysts of *Cryptosporidium baileyi* and *C. galli* [160] and the trophozoites of sleeping sickness (*T. brucei var rhodiense*), leishmaniasis (*L. donovani*) and malaria (*P. vivax*) [158] protozoa. Carvacrol was most potent against *T. brucei var rhodiense* (IC_{50} 0.15 µg/ml) [158]. *L. donovani, P. vivax* [158] and *L. infantum* [159] displayed less sensitivity to carvacrol (IC_{50} of 6.4, 13.1 and 9.8 µg/ml, respectively). Hamsters treated with carvacrol (100 mg/kg/injection) seven days after *L. infantum* infection displayed reduced liver damage and parasite burden compared with a control group [159]. Carvacrol's anti-leishmanial activity has been attributed to an unblocked OH [158] or phenol group with eugenol displaying strong activity (IC_{50} 25-83 µg/ml) against *L. amazonensis* promastigotes [241]. Carvacrol added to *in vitro* cultures of *Melodogyne incognita* nematode eggs (250 mg/L) [161] or mixed into soil containing nematodes (75-100 mg/kg) [161, 242], decreased both their viability and their ability to form galls on tomato [161] or cucumber plants [242].

Antiviral

Carvacrol has been reported to display activity against at least eight viruses [152 - 155, 214, 216, 243]. Several mechanisms of action have been identified that impair penetration or replication of bovine viral diarrhea virus [243], SARS-Co--2 [153], HIV [152], HPV-1 [155, 211], HPV-2 [216], norovirus [154], respiratory syncytial virus [243] and rotavirus [243].

Semi-synthetic Analogs of Carvacrol

Seven literature studies have reported the creation of analogs of carvacrol and tested them against either bacteria [182, 245 - 248], fungi [247, 248], protozoa

[249] or helminths [250] (Table **3**). The majority have investigated antibacterial

Table 3. ***In vitro*** **antimicrobial effects of carvacrol.**

Analogs Created	**Results**	**References**
Carvacrol methyl ether, carvacryl acetate	↑ activity against gram-positive and gram-negative bacteria (MIC >3 mg/ml). Similar data for two fungi.	[182]
Seven ester forms of carvacrol	↑ activity against *B. subtilis*, *E. coli*, *S. aureus* and *S. mutans* (MIC 23 to > 1,000 µg/ml); curcumin (MIC 11.7-23.4 µg ml).	[245]
Four analogs (2- and 4-ally-, propyl- and methylallyl)	↑ activity against *P. aeruginosa* and *S. epidermidis* planktonic forms (MIC 23 to > 1,000 µg/ml). ↓ BEC ($p<0.05$) of 2-allyl (9.25 mM) and 4- allyl (3.25 mM) derivatives.	[246]
Twenty-three analogs of carvacrol created using 4 schemes	Three (hydrophilic) equivalent to carvacrol against gram-negative bacteria, two were antifungal and one more effective against *Candida* sp. than carvacrol.	[247]
Ten analogs carvacrol OH group to carboxyl sulfur amino acids	Evaluated against 4 bacteria and *C. albicans*. One antibacterial (MIC 2.5 mg/ml) for all bacteria except *P. aeruginosa* (MIC 5 mg/ml). ↓ *E. coli* biofilms. Good activity against *C. albicans* (MIC 0.3-2.5 mg/ml).	[248]
Ortho-, meta- and para-nitro MBHA analogs of carvacrol	*L. amazonensis* promastigotes. All three analogs were significantly ($p<0.05$) more potent (IC_{50} 13-22 µM) compared with the parent carvacrol (IC_{50} 138 µM).	[249]
Carvacryl acetate (CA)	CA less potent than carvacrol at preventing egg hatching of *Haemonchus contortus* (EC_{50} 1.7 mg/ml and 0.17 mg/m, respectively).	[250]
Carvacryl acetate (CA)	CA 6.25 µg/ml ↓ *S. mansoni* motility and doses less than this ↓ egg viability and output.	[251]

Abbreviations: BEC (biofilm eradicating concentration), EC_{50} (half maximal inhibitory concentration for egg hatching), h (hour), IC_{50} (half maximal inhibitory concentration), LD_{50} (lethal dose for 50% of animals), MHBA (Morita-Bayliss-Hillman adduct), MIC (minimum inhibitory concentration).

activities [182, 245 - 248]. Two studies concluded that blocking the OH group by either acetylation [182] or esterification [245], significantly reduced antibacterial activity. Simple allyl group substitutions (2- or 4-allyl carvacrol) significantly increased ($p<0.05$) carvacrol antibacterial activity against both gram-positive (*S. epidermidis*) and gram-negative (*P. aeruginosa*) bacteria [246]. Walsh *et al.* [246] reported a hierarchy of antibacterial efficacy for their carvacrol analogs of 2- and 4-allyl> carvacrol>2-methallyl>2-*n*-propyl carvacrol. BEC of *P. aeruginosa* and *S. epidermidis* biofilms was several-fold higher for 2-allyl and 4-allyl carvacrol than carvacrol [246]. Cacciatore *et al.* [247] reported similar antibacterial data for an allyl-cysteine substituted carvacrol (*N*-Ac-Cys(Allyl)-CAR) against planktonic strains of *E. coli*, *S. aureus* and *S. epidermidis*. These authors also confirmed that the allyl-carvacrol was weaker at dissociating *P. aeruginosa* and *S. epidermidis* biofilms but reported it was able to remove those of *E. coli* (biofilm inhibitory concentration BIC 20 mg/ml) compared with carvacrol (BIC 40 mg/ml) [247].

Marinelli *et al.* [248] created three hydrophilic bipartite analogs (WSCP 1-3) by conjugating the hydroxyl group of carvacrol directly to the carboxylic acid group of either glycine or alanine, displayed similar potencies against gram-negative bacteria (MIC range 64-256 μg/ml) [248]. Carvacrol analogs created using 3,3 dimethyl allyl chloride (WSCP 18) or geranyl chloride (WSCP19), were ineffective against gram-negative bacteria but significantly better ($p<0.05$) against *S. pneumoniae* (MIC 64 and 16 μg/ml, respectively) and *E. faecalis* (MIC 128 μg/ml and 64 μg/ml, respectively) than carvacrol (256 μg/ml) [248]. None of these five agents were toxic to human keratinocytes, *in vitro* [248].

Cacciatore *et al.* [247] and Marinelli *et al.* [248] investigated the antifungal effects of their carvacrol analogs on *Candida* species. Three of the Cacciatore *et al.* [247] analogs were as effective against *C. albicans* (MIC 0.3, 0.15 and 0.5 mg/ml, respectively) as carvacrol (MIC 0.3 mg/ml). WSCP1 was more effective against *Candida* sp. (MIC 0.8 mg/ml) than carvacrol (MIC 1.25 mg/ml) [248]. One study of *o*, *m*- and *p*-nitro adducts of carvacrol (MHBA-CAR) identified that these displayed a more than 10-fold increase in potency *versus* the parent compound [249]. Xavier *et al.* [249] reported the nitrated ortho form was superior (IC_{50} 13.6 μM) than the meta and para forms (IC_{50} 18 and 22 μM). These authors theorized that structure of the ortho MHBA-CAR results in a longer duration of potency against the leishmania membrane [249]. Carvacryl acetate, although ineffective as an antibacterial agent [182], possesses potent anti-helmintic activity against *S. mansoni* [250] and, to a lesser extent, gastrointestinal nematodes [251].

Nanoparticle and Immobilized Carvacrol Studies

Fifteen studies have reported stabilization of antibacterial, antifungal and anti-helminthic activities of carvacrol [176 - 179, 252 - 262] (Table **4**). NP strategies were the most popular method used with nine of the studies investigating carvacrol alone [176, 178, 179, 253, 255, 256, 262], in combination with zinc oxide [177] or in combination with its analog carvacryl acetate [261]. Most studies focused on generating novel antibiotic products [176 - 179, 252 - 259] and reported favorable antibacterial activity against gram-positive [176 - 179, 252 - 254, 256 - 259], or gram-negative bacteria [177 - 179, 255 - 257, 259]. Rao *et al.* [256] evaluated the effect of pH on the antibacterial functionality of their ovalbumin-carvacrol nanoparticles (OCGn-2). At lower pH (pH 2) structure, encapsulation rate and bacteriostatic rate of OCGN-2 were optimal, providing significantly lower ($p<0.05$) MIC against *S. aureus* and *E. coli* than unbound carvacrol [256]. Carvacrol release from functionalized surfaces was measured in four studies with sustained bioavailability reported for at least 2 days [255], 6 days [251], 30 days [176] and, in one study, for more than two months [259].

Using mesoporous MCM-41 microparticles of carvacrol, Bernados *et al.* [260] reported potent, prolonged (up to 30 days) *in vitro* activity against *A. niger*. These authors suggest that the porosity of these NP allowed an even binding of the carvacrol with MCM-41 producing a homogeneous distribution [260]. Gharbi *et al.* [257] created two new molecules, to separate the carvacrol OH from the gold surface and thereby increase antifungal reactivity [261]. Carvacrol acetate showed optimal encapsulation activity and a longer duration of anti-helminthic potency against *in vitro* nematodes but was less effective than carvacrol [262]. This analog has been previously demonstrated to damage the flatworm *S. mansoni* [250, 251].

Table 4. Antimicrobial activity of nanoparticle (NP) and immobilized carvacrol.

In vitro Study Design	Results	References
Chitosan particles, two step method (4-80 nm)	Antibacterial: *S. aureus, B. cereus* and *E. coli* (MIC 0.257 mg/ml).	[176]
Zinc oxide (ZnO) NP	*C. jejuni*; Synergistic effect ~5 log CFU/ml ↓ after 8 h.	[177]
Solid nanoparticles loaded with GMS and PGMP (633 nm);	Antibacterial: *E. coli* 0157: H7 and *S. aureus* (MIC 125 and 100 μg/ml, respectively). Release >30 days.	[178]
PEI-coated PLA carvacrol nanoparticles	Antibacterial: *E. coli, S. enterica, L. monocytogenes* and *S. aureus* (MIC 128-256 μg/ml) Release >6 days.	[179]
PLA fibers- BCNW	Antibacterial: *L. monocytogenes* (DDA 39 mm).	[252]
PLGA carvacrol nanoparticles (10%)	Antibacterial: significant ↓ of pre-formed *S. epidermis* biofilm	[253]
PONI polymers cross-linked to carvacrol	Antibacterial:10% dose significant ↓ of pre-formed biofilms within 3 h.	[254]
PHB NP	Antibacterial: *E. coli.*	[255]
OCGns created using pH ranges 2-9; pH 2 optimal	Antibacterial: *B. cereus* (MIC 0.08 mg/ml), Salmonella (MIC 0.16 mg/ml).	[256]
Polymer carvacrol/ palygorskite clay	Antibacterial: *S. aureus* and *E. coli.* Non-toxic to human fibroblasts.	[257]
Cellulose nanocrystals β-CD derivatization	Antibacterial: *B. cereus* and prolonged carvacrol release (2 days).	[258]
Bio-bed, cross-linked material, diffusion-controlled system (20% carvacrol)	Antibacterial: *S. aureus* and *E. coli* prolonged carvacrol release (>2 months) ↓ adhesion of 100% and 98%, respectively.	[259]

(Table 4) cont.....

In vitro Study Design	Results	References
MCM-41 and β-CD microparticles (2.29 nm)	Antifungal: MCM-41↓ *A. fumigatus* significantly ($p<0.05$) by 15 days.	[260]
Gold surface with ester bond functionalized	Antifungal: *C. albicans* ↓ viability by 65% during 3 h culture.	[261]
Chitosan nanoparticles, bilayer system with CVA (500 nm)	Anti-helminthic: *Haemonchus contortus* (IC_{50} 150 ng/ml, 6 h).	[262]

Abbreviations: BCNW (bacterial cellulose nanowhiskers), β-CD (β-cyclodextrin), CFU = colony forming units, CVA (carvacryl Acetate), DDA (disc diffusion assay) GMS (glyceryl monostearate), h = hours, MCM-41 (Mobil Composition of Matter No. 41), MIC (minimum inhibitory concentration), OCGn (ovalbumin-carvacrol nanoparticle), PEI (polythethylenemine), PGMP (propylene glycol monopalmitate), PHB (polyhydroxybutyrate), PLA (polylactate), PLGA (Poly(DL-lactide-co-glycolide), PONI (poly(oxanorborneneimide).

NP carvacrol also potentiates other antimicrobial agents [177, 260, 263 - 266]. Combination of carvacrol with cinnaminaldehyde [264], eugenol [263, 264], and thymol [265] was as effective as pharmaceutical agents against both planktonic gram-positive [264, 265] and gram-negative [263 - 265] bacteria, *in vitro*. Windiasti *et al.* [177] reported that carvacrol damaged *C. jejuni* membranes allowing zinc oxide to induce cell leakage and lysis. Engel *et al.* [265] reported thymol and carvacrol liposomes could disperse early stage of *S. enterica* and *S. aureus* biofilms within 10 minutes of exposure.

DISCUSSION AND FUTURE DIRECTIONS

This chapter has described at least 13 effective bioavailable analogs and 22 nanoparticle or stabilized derivatives of allicin and carvacrol [80, 126 - 129, 131 - 137, 176 - 179, 182, 245 - 250]. For any of these agents to become pharmaceutical products would require them to go through a lengthy and costly Food and Drug Administration (FDA) approval process [266, 267]. Current estimates are that around 12% of all candidate molecules become medications, with 60% failing as they are not sufficiently selective for their target, prove toxic or are ineffective in humans [267]. A final issue is purity and stability, as many potent biological molecules also have short half-lives [268]. One alternative is to focus on developing topical agents, which are required by the FDA only to prove non-irritant and non-toxic if ingested [267]. Allicin and carvacrol are naturally non-toxic or have safe created derivatives [32, 169]. Allicin and carvacrol stabilized preparations were created using safe materials [131 - 137, 176 - 179, 252 - 262]. Analogs and NP derivatives of carvacrol in particular are stable for days [251, 255] or months [17, 259, 260] and in these forms are pure and reproducible.

Topical Agents

Although topically applied pharmaceutical products constitute less than one in ten of all new pharmaceuticals [266], allicin and carvacrol derivatives could be feasible as antifungal agents [131, 260, 261] to treat multi-resistant, biofilm-forming skin bacterial infections [89, 90, 135, 219, 220, 246, 253] and even for some protozoa *e.g.* Leishmaniasis [158 - 160, 249]. Dermatophyte infections are common and in need of novel interventions given current limited strategies [19, 20]. Novel treatments may come from creams containing nanoparticle-coupled allicin [131, 135, 136].

Novel Drug Candidates

Pharmaceutical industries are also searching for novel drug candidates that interfere with important antimicrobial pathways [1, 2]. Several lead molecules suggest themselves [153, 216]. Synthetic allicin inhibits early phase reproductive genes for HCMV [77], carvacrol can bind to the major protease (M^{pro}) for SARS-CoV2 preventing its replication [154] and decrease viral gene expression in HSV-2 [213]. New anti-helminthic drugs might also come from NP or microemulsion formulations of carvacrol or carvacrol acetate [250, 251, 262].

Combinatorial Therapies

Allicin [87] and carvacrol [156, 221, 228 - 230, 232] both potentiate the *in vitro* effects of current antibiotics and antifungal medications significantly decreasing the doses needed for efficacy. Carvacrol NP are important adjuncts to removing pre-formed [246, 248] bacterial biofilms [247, 249] and could be used alone or to potentiate antibiotics. Certainly, NP containing silver, gold or zinc oxide combined with allicin [135, 136] or carvacrol [177, 261] have been demonstrated to be effective antibacterial agents. Valcourt *et al.* [264] reported a combined NP composed of doxycycline, carvacrol, eugenol and cinnaminaldehyde significantly increased the efficacy of the antibiotic, reducing its MIC against five gram-negative species 4-fold.

Packaging Materials

Several studies have successfully developed carvacrol as a surface treatment that might be used as packaging agents to prevent food spoilage [258, 259, 270]. De Castro *et al.* [270] recently created a bonded cellulose medium that was able to significantly ($p<0.05$) and consistently release a combination of carvacrol and curcumin to and eliminate bacteria over a 24-hour period.

Fish and Animal Agents

Resistance to antifungal and antibacterial treatments is more than an issue for humans, it also affects the food supplies of millions [23, 104 - 107, 271].

Helminths and nematodes are a particular issue with few effective interventions in preventing farmed animal weight loss and demise [259]. Significant and rapid efficacy has been demonstrated *in vitro* by the carvacrol analog carvacryl acetate against *S. mansoni* [247] and chitosan carvacrol-NP against *H. contortus* [259]. These certainly provide good lead entities for future research.

Final Thoughts

Our process of discovering new antimicrobials has changed significantly since the discover of penicillin in 1928 [12]. An understanding of the scope of activity of natural phytochemicals can now be coupled with new biochemical and physical chemical strategies to create novel moieties with activities matching or bettering current agents. To avoid the cycle of resistance driving new design some researchers now argue for the natural molecular approach [9, 12, 15 - 17]. It is to be anticipated that allicin and carvacrol, in all their newly created forms will be a part of this process.

CONSENT FOR PUBLICATION

Not Applicable.

CONFLICT OF INTEREST

The author confirms that this chapter contents have no conflict of interest.

ACKNOWLDEGEMENTS

Thanks go to Dr. Kathryn Mickle for the preparation of figure 1 in this manuscript.

REFERENCES

[1] Pan S-Y, Litscher G, Gao S-H, *et al.* Historical perspective of traditional indigenous medical practices: the current renaissance and conservation of herbal resources. Evid Based Complement Alternat Med 2014; 2014: 525340. [cited 6th December 2020]. [http://dx.doi.org/10.1155/2014/525340] [PMID: 24872833]

[2] Folashade O, Omoregie H, Ochogu P. Standardization of herbal medicines-A review. Int J Biodivers Conserv 2012; 4: 101-12.https://academicjournals.org/journal/IJBC/article-full-text-pdf/B1481FE9709 [cited 6th December 2020].

[3] Solecki RS. Shanidar IV, a Neanderthal flower burial in Northern Iraq. Science 1975; 190(4217): 880-1. [http://dx.doi.org/10.1126/science.190.4217.880]

[4] Petrovska BB. Historical review of medicinal plants' usage. Pharmacogn Rev 2012; 6(11): 1-5.

[5] Dorofeeva-Lichtmann VV. Conception of Terrestrial Organization in the Shan Hai Jing. Bulletin De L'École Française D'Extrême-Orient 1995; 82: 57-110.www.jstor.org/stable/43730894 [http://dx.doi.org/10.3406/befeo.1995.2297]

[6] Hintz T, Matthews KK, Di R. The use of plant antimicrobial compounds for food preservation. BioMed Res Int 2015; 2015: 246264. [cited 6th December 2020].
[http://dx.doi.org/10.1155/2015/246264] [PMID: 26539472]

[7] Dorman HJD, Deans SG. Antimicrobial agents from plants: antibacterial activity of plant volatile oils. Journal of Applied Microbiology 88: 308-16.
[http://dx.doi.org/10.1046/j.1365-2672.2000.00969.x]

[8] Cowan MM. Plant products as antimicrobial agents. Clin Microbiol Rev 1999; 12(4): 564-82. https://www.ncbi.nlm.nih.gov/pmc/articles/PMC88925/ [cited 6th December 2020].
[http://dx.doi.org/10.1128/CMR.12.4.564] [PMID: 10515903]

[9] Hu Q, Zhou M, Wei S. Progress on the Antimicrobial Activity Research of Clove Oil and Eugenol in the Food Antisepsis Field. J Food Sci 2018; 83(6): 1476-83. [cited 6th December 2020].
[http://dx.doi.org/10.1111/1750-3841.14180] [PMID: 29802735]

[10] Sharifi-Rad M, Varoni EM, Iriti M, *et al.* Carvacrol and human health: A comprehensive review. Phytother Res 2018; 32(9): 1675-87.
[http://dx.doi.org/10.1002/ptr.6103]

[11] Maia MF, Moore SJ. Plant-based insect repellents: a review of their efficacy, development and testing. Malar J 2011; 10(Suppl 1): S11.
[http://dx.doi.org/10.1186/1475-2875-10-S1-S11]

[12] Veeresham C. Natural products derived from plants as a source of drugs. J Adv Pharm Technol Res 2012; 3(4): 200-1.
[http://dx.doi.org/10.4103/2231-4040.104709]

[13] Saga T, Yamaguchi K. Natural products derived from plants as a source of drugs. J Adv Pharm Technol Res 2009; 3(4): 200-1. http://www.med.or.jp/english/pdf/2009_02/103_108.pdf

[14] Updahyay A, Upadhyaya I, Kollanor-Johny A, Venikanraranan K. Combatting pathogenic microorganisms using plant-derived antimicrobials: A minireview of the mechanistic basis. BioMed Res Int 2014; 761741.
[http://dx.doi.org/10.1155/2014/761741]

[15] Cundell DR. Herbal Medicines as Immunomodulators. Curr Immunol Rev 2014; 10(2): 64-81.
http://www.currentimmunologyreviews.com/articles/124626/herbal-phytochemicals-as-immunomodulators [cited 6th December 2020].
[http://dx.doi.org/10.2174/1573395510666140915213156]

[16] Ventola CL. The antibiotic resistance crisis: part 1: causes and threats. P&T 2015; 40(4): 277-83.https://www.ncbi.nlm.nih.gov/pmc/articles/PMC4378521/ [cited 6th December 2020].
[PMID: 25859123]

[17] Kontoyiannis DP. Antifungal Resistance: An Emerging Reality and A Global Challenge. J Infect Dis 2017; 216(3) (suppl_3): S431-5. [cited 6th December 2020].
[http://dx.doi.org/10.1093/infdis/jix179] [PMID: 28911044]

[18] Koo H, Allan RN, Howlin RP, Stoodley P, Hall-Stoodley L. Targeting microbial biofilms: current and prospective therapeutic strategies. Nat Rev Microbiol 2017; 15(12): 740-55. [cited 7th December 2020].
[http://dx.doi.org/10.1038/nrmicro.2017.99] [PMID: 28944770]

[19] Mpoza E, Rhein J, Abassi M. Emerging fluconazole resistance: Implications for the management of cryptococcal meningitis. Med Mycol Case Rep 2017; 19: 30-2.

[20] Li M, Liao Y, Chen M, Pan W, Weng L. Antifungal susceptibilities of Cryptococcus species complex isolates from AIDS and non-AIDS patients in Southeast China. Braz J Infect Dis 2012; 16(2): 175-9. [cited 7th December 2020].
[http://dx.doi.org/10.1590/S1413-86702012000200012] [PMID: 22552461]

[21] Yenisehirli G, Bulut N, Yenisehirli A, Bulut Y. *In Vitro* Susceptibilities of *Candida albicans* Isolates to Antifungal Agents in Tokat, Turkey. Jundishapur J Microbiol 2015; 8(9): e28057.

[22] Barros MEDS, Santos DA, Hamdan JS. Evaluation of susceptibility of Trichophyton mentagrophytes and Trichophyton rubrum clinical isolates to antifungal drugs using a modified CLSI microdilution method (M38-A). J Med Microbiol 2007; 56(Pt 4): 514-8.

[23] Fisher MC, Hawkins MJ, Sanglard D, Gurr SJ. 2018 Worldwide emergence of resistance to antifungal drugs challenges human health and food security. Science 360: 6390:739-742.

[24] Lee SM, Kim MS, Hayat F, Shin D. Recent Advances in the Discovery of Novel Antiprotozoal Agents. Molecules 2019; 24(21): 3886. [http://dx.doi.org/10.3390/molecules24213886]

[25] Blair W, Cox C. Current Landscape of Antiviral Drug Discovery. F1000Res Faculty Rev-202 2016; 5: F1000.

[26] Leisner JJ. The Diverse Search for Synthetic, Semisynthetic and Natural Product Antibiotics From the 1940s and Up to 1960 Exemplified by a Small Pharmaceutical Player. Frontiers in Microbiology 2020; 11: 976.

[27] Khan RA, Khan RA. Natural products chemistry: The emerging trends and prospective goals. Saudi Pharm J 2018; 26(5): 739-53. [cited 28th February 2021]. [http://dx.doi.org/10.1016/j.jsps.2018.02.015] [PMID: 29991919]

[28] Krishna S, Bustamante L, Haynes RK, Staines HM. Artemisinins: their growing importance in medicine. Trends Pharmacol Sci 2008; 29(10): 520-7. [http://dx.doi.org/10.1016/j.tips.2008.07.004]

[29] Yuan-Chieh Y, Tse-Hung H, Shih-Chun Y, Chin-Chang C, Jia-You F. Nano-Based Drug Delivery or Targeting to Eradicate Bacteria for Infection Mitigation: A Review of Recent Advances. Frontiers in Chemistry 2020; 8: 286.

[30] Sandhiya V, Ubaidulla U. A review on herbal drug loaded into pharmaceutical carrier techniques and its evaluation process. Futur J Pharm Sci 2020; 6: 51. [cited 7th December 2020]. [http://dx.doi.org/10.1186/s43094-020-00050-0]

[31] Block E. *Allium* botany and cultivation, ancient and modern. In: Block E, Ed. Garlic and other alliums: The Lore and the Science. Royal Society of Chemistry 2010.www.rsc.org

[32] Borlinghaus J, Albrecht F, Gruhlke MC, Nwachukwu ID, Slusarenko AJ. Allicin: chemistry and biological properties. Molecules 2014; 19(8): 12591-618. [http://dx.doi.org/10.3390/molecules190812591]

[33] Rahman MS. Allicin and other functional active components in garlic: health benefits and bioavailability. Int J Food Prop 2007; 10: 245-68. [http://dx.doi.org/10.1080/10942910601113327]

[34] Cundell DR. Allicin: history, ethnobotany and uses as told primarily by the garlic plant. In: Cundell DR, Ed. Allicin the Natural Sulfur Compound from Garlic with Many Uses. New York: Nova Science Publishers Inc. 2020; pp. 1-24.

[35] Petrovska BB, Cekovska S. Extracts from the history and medical properties of garlic. Pharmacogn Rev 2010; 4(7): 106-10. [http://dx.doi.org/10.4103/0973-7847.65321] [PMID: 22228949]

[36] Lawson LD. 1998. Garlic a review of its medicinal effects and active compounds. In Phytomedicines of Europe. Chemistry and Biological Activity. Eds. Lawson LD, Bauer R. Washington DC; ACS Symposium Series 691: pp 176-209. [http://dx.doi.org/10.1021/bk-1998-0691.ch014]

[37] Moyers S. Garlic in health, history and world cuisine. St. Petersburg, FL. Suncoast Press 1996; 1996: 1-36.

[38] Cavallito CJ, Bailey JH. Allicin, the antibacterial principle of *Allium sativum*. I. Isolation, physical properties and antibacterial action. J Am Chem Soc 1944; 66: 1950-1. [http://dx.doi.org/10.1021/ja01239a048]

[39] Tsao S-M, Yin M-C. *In-vitro* antimicrobial activity of four diallyl sulphides occurring naturally in garlic and Chinese leek oils. J Med Microbiol 2001; 50(7): 646-9. [http://dx.doi.org/10.1099/0022-1317-50-7-646] [PMID: 11444776]

[40] Satyal P, Craft JD, Dosoky NS. The chemical compositions of the volatile oils of garlic (*Allium sativum*) and wild garlic (*Allium vineale*). Foods 2017; 6(8): 63.

[41] Wagner-Graham MA. A contemporary overview of allicin, an ancient antibiotic. In: Cundell DR, Ed. Allicin the Natural Sulfur Compound from Garlic with Many Uses. New York: Nova Science Publishers Inc. 2020; pp. 111-50.

[42] French-Arthur BM. Antifungal activity of allicin. In: Cundell DR, Ed. Allicin the Natural Sulfur Compound from Garlic with Many Uses. New York: Nova Science Publishers Inc. 2020; pp. 151-68.

[43] French-Arthur BM. Anti-protozoal and anti-helminthic activity of allicin. In: Cundell DR, Ed. Allicin the Natural Sulfur Compound from Garlic with Many Uses. New York: Nova Science Publishers Inc. 2020; pp. 169-86.

[44] Cundell DR. Virucidal activity of allicin. In: Cundell DR, Ed. Allicin the Natural Sulfur Compound from Garlic with Many Uses. New York: Nova Science Publishers Inc. 2020; pp. 187-210.

[45] Li G, Ma X, Deng L, *et al.* Fresh Garlic Extract Enhances the Antimicrobial Activities of Antibiotics on Resistant Strains *in vitro*. Jundishapur J Microbiol 2015; 8(5): e14814.

[46] Kim Y-S, Kim KS, Han I, Kim M-H, Jung MH, Park H-K. Quantitative and qualitative analysis of the antifungal activity of allicin alone and in combination with antifungal drugs. PLoS One 2012; 7(6): e38242.

[47] Gupta KC, Viswanathan R. Combined action of streptomycin and chloramphenicol with plant antibiotics against tubercle bacilli. I. Streptomycin and chloramphenicol with cepharanthine. II. Streptomycin and allicin. Antibiot Chemother (Northfield) 1955; 5(1): 24-7. [PMID: 24543344]

[48] Bachrach G, Jamil A, Naor R, Tal G, Ludmer Z, Steinberg D. Garlic allicin as a potential agent for controlling oral pathogens. J Med Food 2011; 14(11): 1338-43. [http://dx.doi.org/10.1089/jmf.2010.0165] [PMID: 21548800]

[49] Waag T, Gelhaus C, Rath J, Stich A, Leippe M, Schirmeister T. Allicin and derivates are cysteine protease inhibitors with antiparasitic activity. Bioorg Med Chem Lett 2010; 20(18): 5541-3. [http://dx.doi.org/10.1016/j.bmcl.2010.07.062]

[50] Lemar KM, Passa O, Aon MA, *et al.* Allyl alcohol and garlic (*Allium sativum*) extract produce oxidative stress in *Candida albicans* . Microbiology (Reading) 2005; 151(Pt 10): 3257-65.

[51] Focke M, Feld A, Lichtenthaler K. Allicin, a naturally occurring antibiotic from garlic, specifically inhibits acetyl-CoA synthetase. FEBS Lett 1990; 261(1): 106-8. [http://dx.doi.org/10.1016/0014-5793(90)80647-2]

[52] Atkinson HJ, Babbitt PC, Sajid M. The global cysteine peptidase landscape in parasites. Trends Parasitol 2009; 25(12): 573-81. [http://dx.doi.org/10.1016/j.pt.2009.09.006]

[53] Cundell DR, Wilkinson F. Plant Factors inhibitory to biofilm formation.Ebook Biofilms, characterization, applications and recent advances. Nova, NY, USA 2016.

[54] Cady NC, McKean KA, Behnke J, *et al.* Inhibition of biofilm formation, quorum sensing and infection in *Pseudomonas aeruginosa* by natural products-inspired organosulfur compounds. PLoS One 2012; 7(6): e38492. [http://dx.doi.org/10.1371/journal.pone.0038492] [PMID: 22715388]

[55] Cruz-Villalón G, Pérez-Giraldo C. Effect of allicin on the production of polysaccharide intercellular adhesin in *Staphylococcus epidermidis* . J Appl Microbiol 2011; 110(3): 723-8. [http://dx.doi.org/10.1111/j.1365-2672.2010.04929.x] [PMID: 21205098]

[56] Zhai H, Pan J, Pang E, Bai B. Lavage with allicin in combination with vancomycin inhibits biofilm formation by *Staphylococcus epidermidis* in a rabbit model of prosthetic joint infection. PLoS One 2014; 9(7): e102760. [cited 21st November 2020]. [http://dx.doi.org/10.1371/journal.pone.0102760] [PMID: 25025650]

[57] Guan X, Zhou Y, Chen H, Wang C, Wang H. Antibacterial, anti-inflammatory, and anti-osteoclastogenesis roles of allicin in periodontitis. Int J Clin Med 2018; 11(7): 6721-30.http://www.ijcem.com/files/ijcem0066740.pdf [cited 21st November 2020].

[58] Corral MJ, Benito-Peña E, Jiménez-Antón MD, Cuevas L, Moreno-Bondi MC, Alunda JM. Allicin Induces Calcium and Mitochondrial Dysregulation Causing Necrotic Death in Leishmania. PLoS Negl Trop Dis 2016; 10(3): e0004525. [cited 21st November 2020]. [http://dx.doi.org/10.1371/journal.pntd.0004525] [PMID: 27023069]

[59] Ankri S, Miron T, Rabinkov A, Wilchek M, Mirelman D. Allicin from garlic strongly inhibits cysteine proteinases and cytopathic effects of *Entamoeba histolytica.* Antimicrob Agents Chemother 1997; 41(10): 2286-8.

[60] Argüello-García R, de la Vega-Arnaud M, Loredo-Rodríguez IJ, *et al.* Activity of Thioallyl Compounds From Garlic Against Giardia duodenalis Trophozoites and in Experimental Giardiasis. Front Cell Infect Microbiol 2018; 8: 353.

[61] Coppi A, Cabinian M, Mirelman D, Sinnis P. Antimalarial activity of allicin, a biologically active compound from garlic cloves. Antimicrob Agents Chemother 2006; 50(5): 1731-7. [http://dx.doi.org/10.1128/AAC.50.5.1731-1737.2006]

[62] Feng Y, Zhu X, Wang Q, *et al.* Allicin enhances host pro-inflammatory immune responses and protects against acute murine malaria infection. Malar J 2012; 11: 268. [cited 27th November 2020]. [http://dx.doi.org/10.1186/1475-2875-11-268] [PMID: 22873687]

[63] Borjihan H, Ogita A, Fujita K, Hirasawa E, Tanaka T. The vacuole-targeting fungicidal activity of amphotericin B against the pathogenic fungus *Candida albicans* and its enhancement by allicin. J Antibiot (Tokyo) 2009; 62(12): 691-7.

[64] Alouf JE, Stephen J, Billington SJ, Jost BH. Repertoir and general features of the family of cholesterol-dependent cytolysins. The Comprehensive Sourcebook of Bacterial Protein Toxins. Eds. Alouf and Popoff. Elsevier Ltd. 2006; pp. 643-8. [http://dx.doi.org/10.1016/B978-012088445-2/50041-X]

[65] Arzanlou M, Bohlooli S. Inhibition of streptolysin O by allicin - an active component of garlic. J Med Microbiol 2010; 59(Pt 9): 1044-9.

[66] Arzanlou M, Bohlooli S, Jannati E, Mirzanejad-Asl H. Allicin from garlic neutralizes the hemolytic activity of intra- and extra-cellular pneumolysin O *in vitro*. Toxicon 2011; 57(4): 540-5.

[67] Leng B-F, Qiu J-Z, Dai X-H, *et al.* Allicin reduces the production of α-toxin by *Staphylococcus aureus* . Molecules 2011; 16(9): 7958-68. [http://dx.doi.org/10.3390/molecules16097958] [PMID: 21921868]

[68] Ranjbar-Omid M, Arzanlou M, Amani M, *et al.* Allicin from garlic inhibits the biofilm formation and urease activity of *Proteus mirabilis in vitro*. FEMS Microbiology Letters 2015; 362(9): fnv049.

[69] Sarfraz M, Nasim MJ, Jacob C, Gruhlke MCH. Efficacy of Allicin against Plant Pathogenic Fungi and Unveiling the Underlying Mode of Action Employing Yeast Based Chemogenetic Profiling Approach. Appl Sci 2020; 10: 2563.

[70] Feldberg RS, Chang SC, Kotik AN, *et al.* *In vitro* mechanism of inhibition of bacterial cell growth by allicin. Antimicrob Agents Chemother 1988; 32(12): 1763-8.

[http://dx.doi.org/10.1128/AAC.32.12.1763] [PMID: 2469386]

[71] Prager-Khoutorsky M, Goncharov I, Rabinkov A, Mirelman D, Geiger B, Bershadsky AD. Allicin inhibits cell polarization, migration and division *via* its direct effect on microtubules. Cell Motil Cytoskeleton 2007; 64(5): 321-7.

[72] Fawzi EM, Elseohaby I. Prevalence of gastrointestinal nematodes and the role of allicin in treatment of cattle in Sharkia governorate. Zagazig Veterinary Journal 2018; 45(1): 109-17. [cited 27th November 2020].
[http://dx.doi.org/10.21608/zvjz.2019.28655]

[73] Borjihan H, Ogita A, Fujita K, Hirasawa E, Tanaka T. The vacuole-targeting fungicidal activity of amphotericin B against the pathogenic fungus *Candida albicans* and its enhancement by allicin. J Antibiot (Tokyo) 2009; 62(12): 691-7. [cited 26th November 2020].
[http://dx.doi.org/10.1038/ja.2009.103] [PMID: 19876074]

[74] Khodavandi A, Alizadeh F, Harmal NS, *et al.* Comparison between efficacy of allicin and fluconazole against *Candida albicansin vitro* and in a systemic candidiasis mouse model. FEMS Microbiol Lett 2011; 315(2): 87-93. [cited 26th November 2020].
[http://dx.doi.org/10.1111/j.1574-6968.2010.02170.x] [PMID: 21204918]

[75] Khodavandi A, Alizadeh F, Aala F, Sekawi Z, Chong PP. *In vitro* investigation of antifungal activity of allicin alone and in combination with azoles against *Candida* species. Mycopathologia 2010; 169(4): 287-95. [cited 26th November 2020].
[http://dx.doi.org/10.1007/s11046-009-9251-3] [PMID: 19924565]

[76] Mehrbod P, Amini E, Tavassoti-Kheiri M. Antiviral activity of garlic extract on influenza virus. Iranian J Virology 2009; 3(1): 19-23. https://www.sid.ir/en/journal/ViewPaper.aspx?ID=168987
[http://dx.doi.org/10.21859/isv.3.1.19]

[77] Fang F, Li H, Cui W, Dong Y. Treatment of hepatitis caused by cytomegalovirus with allitridin injection--an experimental study. J Tongji Med Univ 1999; 19(4): 271-4. [cited 28th November 2020].
[http://dx.doi.org/10.1007/BF02886960] [PMID: 12938515]

[78] Casini A, Scozzafava A, Claudiu Supuran C. Cysteine-modifying agents: a possible effective approach for antiviral and anticancer drugs. Environmental Health Perspectives 2002; 110(5): 801-6.
[http://dx.doi.org/10.1289/ehp.02110s5801]

[79] Coppi A, Natarajan R, Pradel G, *et al.* The malaria circumsporozoite protein has two functional domains, each with distinct roles as sporozoites journey from mosquito to mammalian host. J Exp Med 2011; 208(2): 341-56.

[80] Sunil S, Chauhan VS, Malhotra P. Distinct and stage specific nuclear factors regulate the expression of falcipains, *Plasmodium falciparum* cysteine proteases. BMC Mol Biol 2008;9: 47.

[81] Lima CMBL, Freitas FIS, Morais LC, *et al.* Ultrastructural study on the morphological changes to male worms of *Schistosoma mansoni* after *in vitro* exposure to allicin. Rev Soc Bras Med Trop 2011; 44(3): 327-30. http://www.scielo.br/scielo.php?script=sci_arttext&pid=S0037-86822011000300013&lng=en [cited 27th November 2020].
[http://dx.doi.org/10.1590/S0037-86822011005000023] [PMID: 21537796]

[82] Wang Q, Da'dara AA, Skelly PJ. The human blood parasite *Schistosoma mansoni* expresses extracellular tegumental calpains that cleave the blood clotting protein fibronectin. Sci Rep 2017;7(1):12912.

[83] Bakri IM, Douglas CW. Inhibitory effect of garlic extract on oral bacteria. Archives of Oral Biology 200; 50 (7): 645-651.
[http://dx.doi.org/10.1016/j.archoralbio.2004.12.002]

[84] Berube BJ, Bubeck Wardenburg J. *Staphylococcus aureus* α-toxin: nearly a century of intrigue. Toxins (Basel) 2013;5(6):1140-1166.

[85] Tan L, Rui LS, Bei J, Mei HX, Shu L. Therapeutic targeting of the *Staphylococcus aureus* accessory

gene regulator (agr) system. Frontiers in Microbiology 2018; 9: 55.

[86] National Center for Biotechnology Information (2020). PubChem Compound Summary for CID 2082, Albendazole. Retrieved 28th November 2020. https://pubchem.ncbi.nlm.nih.gov/compound/Albendazole

[87] Reiter J, Levina N, van der Linden M, Gruhlke M, Martin C, Slusarenko AJ. Diallylthiosulfinate (allicin), a volatile antimicrobial from garlic (*Allium sativum*), kills human lung pathogenic bacteria, including MDR strains, as a vapor. Molecules 2017; 22(10): 1711. [http://dx.doi.org/10.3390/molecules22101711] [PMID: 29023413]

[88] Kulik EM, Thurnheer T, Karygianni L, Walter C, Sculean A, Eick S. Antibiotic Susceptibility Patterns of *Aggregatibacter actinomycetemcomitans* and *Porphyromonas gingivalis* Strains from Different Decades. Antibiotics (Basel). 2019;8(4):253.

[89] Cutler RR, Wilson P. Antibacterial activity of a new, stable, aqueous extract of allicin against methicillin-resistant *Staphylococcus aureus* . Br J Biomed Sci 2004; 61(2): 71-4. [http://dx.doi.org/10.1080/09674845.2004.11732646] [PMID: 15250668]

[90] Tsao SM, Hsu CC, Yin MC. Garlic extract and two diallyl sulphides inhibit methicillin-resistant *Staphylococcus aureus* infection in BALB/cA mice. J Antimicrob Chemother 2003; 52(6): 974-80. [http://dx.doi.org/10.1093/jac/dkg476] [PMID: 14585852]

[91] Jonkers D, Sluimer J, Stobberingh E. Effect of garlic on vancomycin-resistant *enterococci.* Antimicrob Agents Chemother 1999; 43(12): 3045-5. [http://dx.doi.org/10.1128/AAC.43.12.3045] [PMID: 10651625]

[92] Hannan A, Ikram Ullah M, Usman M, Hussain S, Absar M, Javed K. Anti-mycobacterial activity of garlic (*Allium sativum*) against multi-drug resistant and non-multi-drug resistant *mycobacterium tuberculosis.* Pak J Pharm Sci 2011; 24(1): 81-5. [PMID: 21190924]

[93] Ankri S, Mirelman D. Antimicrobial properties of allicin from garlic. Microbes Infect 1999; 1(2): 125-9. [http://dx.doi.org/10.1016/S1286-4579(99)80003-3] [PMID: 10594976]

[94] Roman L, Hohaus N, Jacob C, Gruhlke MHC, Slusarenko AJ. A comparison of the antibacterial and antifungal activities of thiosulfinate analogues of allicin. Sci Rep 2018; 8(1): 1-19. [PMID: 29311619]

[95] Yehia HM, Al-Olayan EM, El-Khadragy MF, Metwally DM. *In vitro* and *in vivo* control of secondary bacterial infection caused by *Leishmania major.* Int J Environ Res Public Health 2017; 14(7): 777. [cited 23rd November 2020]. [http://dx.doi.org/10.3390/ijerph14070777] [PMID: 28703780]

[96] Elsom GK. An antibacterial assay of aqueous extract of garlic against anaerobic/microaerophilic and aerobic bacteria, Microbial Ecology in Health and Disease 2000; 12:2, 81-84.

[97] Wallock-Richards D, Doherty CJ, Doherty L, *et al.* Garlic revisited: antimicrobial activity of allicin-containing garlic extracts against Burkholderia cepacia complex. PLoS One 2014;9(12):e112726.

[98] Borlinghaus J, Bolger A, Schier C, Vogel A, Gruhlke MCH, Slusarenko AJ. Plant-microbe co-evolution: allicin resistance in a *Pseudomonas fluorescens* strain (PfAR-1) isolated from garlic. bioRxiv 2019;769265.

[99] Sitaraman R. Pseudomonas spp. as models for plant-microbe interactions. Front Plant Sci 2015; 6:787.

[100] Baldermann C, Lupas A, Lubieniecki J, Engelhardt H. The regulated outer membrane protein Omp21 from *Comamonas acidovorans* is identified as a member of a new family of eight-stranded beta-sheet proteins by its sequence and properties. J Bacteriol 1998; 180(15): 3741-3749.

[101] Brooke JS. *Stenotrophomonas maltophilia*: an emerging global opportunistic pathogen. Clin Microbiol Rev 2012; 25(1): 2-41.

[http://dx.doi.org/10.1128/CMR.00019-11]

[102] Decker CF, Simon GL, Keiser JF. *Flavimonas oryzihabitans* (*Pseudomonas oryzihabitans*; CDC group Ve-2) bacteremia in the immunocompromised host. Arch Intern Med 1991; 151(3): 603-4. [http://dx.doi.org/10.1001/archinte.1991.00400030133026] [PMID: 2001143]

[103] Llop PL. Genetic islands in pome fruit pathogenic and non-pathogenic Erwinia species and related plasmids. Frontiers in Microbiology 2015; 6:874. [http://dx.doi.org/10.3389/fmicb.2015.00874]

[104] Cundell DR. Allicin and our changing world. In: Cundell DR, Ed. Allicin the Natural Sulfur Compound from Garlic with Many Uses. New York: Nova Science Publishers Inc. 2020; pp. 187-210.

[105] Pu H, Li X, Du Q, Cui H, Xu Y. Research Progress in the Application of Chinese Herbal Medicines in Aquaculture: A Review. Engineering 2017; 3(5): 731-737. [http://dx.doi.org/10.1016/J.ENG.2017.03.017]

[106] Luo QH. Masters Thesis. Effect of the combined food additive Eucommia extract and allicin on the immunity and performance of grass carp. 2008.https://www.globethesis.com/?t=2143360218954062

[107] Nya EJ, Dawood Z, Austin B. The garlic component, allicin, prevents disease caused by *Aeromonas hydrophila* in rainbow trout, *Oncorhynchus mykiss* (Walbaum). J Fish Dis 2010; 33(4): 293-300. [cited 26th November 2020]. [http://dx.doi.org/10.1111/j.1365-2761.2009.01121.x] [PMID: 20082660]

[108] Yamada Y, Azuma K. Evaluation of the *in vitro* antifungal activity of allicin. Antimicrob Agents Chemother 1977; 11(4): 743-9. [http://dx.doi.org/10.1128/AAC.11.4.743] [PMID: 856026]

[109] Davis LE, Shen J, Royer RE. *In vitro* synergism of concentrated *Allium sativum* extract and amphotericin B against *Cryptococcus neoformans* . Planta Med 1994; 60(6): 546-9.

[110] Shadkchan Y, Shemesh E, Mirelman D, *et al.* Efficacy of allicin, the reactive molecule of garlic, in inhibiting Aspergillus spp. *in vitro*, and in a murine model of disseminated aspergillosis. J Antimicrob Chemother 2004; 53(5): 832-6. [http://dx.doi.org/10.1093/jac/dkh174] [PMID: 15044429]

[111] Curtis H, Noll U, Störmann J, Slusarenko AJ. Broad-spectrum Activity of the Volatile Phytoanticipin Allicin in Extracts of Garlic (*Allium Sativum* L.) against Plant Pathogenic Bacteria, Fungi and Oomycetes. Physiol Mol Plant Pathol 2004; 65(2): 79-89. [http://dx.doi.org/10.1016/j.pmpp.2004.11.006]

[112] Parvu M, Barbu-Tudoran L, Rosca-Casian O, Vlase L. Ultrastructural Changes in *Fusarium Oxysporum* F. Sp. Tulipae Hyphae Treated *in vitro* with *Allium Fistulosum* Plant Extract. Annals of the Romanian Society for Cell Biology 2010; 15(2): 65-72.

[113] Mirelman D, Monheit D, Varon S. Inhibition of growth of *Entamoeba histolytica* by allicin, the active principle of garlic extract (*Allium sativum*). J Infect Dis 1987; 156(1): 243-4. [cited 27th November 2020]. [http://dx.doi.org/10.1093/infdis/156.1.243] [PMID: 2885381]

[114] Jesús Corral-Caridad M, Moreno I, Toraño A, Domínguez M, Alunda JM. Effect of allicin on promastigotes and intracellular amastigotes of *Leishmania donovani* and *L. infantum*. Exp Parasitol 2012; 132(4):475-82.

[115] Corral MJ, Serrano DR, Moreno I, Torrado JJ, Domínguez M, Alunda JM. Efficacy of low doses of amphotericin B plus allicin against experimental visceral leishmaniasis. J Antimicrob Chemother. 2014 69(12):3268-74.

[116] Metwally DM, Al-Olayan EM, Alanazi M, Alzahrany SB, Semlali A. Antischistosomal and anti-inflammatory activity of garlic and allicin compared with that of praziquantel *in vivo*. BMC Complement Altern Med 2018; 18(1): 135. [cited 27th November 2020]. [http://dx.doi.org/10.1186/s12906-018-2191-z] [PMID: 29703259]

[117] Gupta R, Sharmaj NK. A study of the nematicidal activity of allicin—an active principle in garlic, *Allium sativum* L., against root-knot nematode, *Meloidogyne incognita* (Kofoid and White, 1919) Chitwood, 1949. International Journal of Pest Management 1993; 39:4, 390-392.

[118] Zhang J, Wang H, Xiang ZD, Shu SN, Fang F. Allitridin inhibits human cytomegalovirus replication *in vitro*. Mol Med Rep 2013; 7(4): 1343-9. [cited 28th November 2020]. [http://dx.doi.org/10.3892/mmr.2013.1328] [PMID: 23426791]

[119] Weber ND, Andersen DO, North JA, Murray BK, Lawson LD, Hughes BG. *In vitro* virucidal effects of *Allium sativum* (garlic) extract and compounds. Planta Med. 1992; 58(5):417-23.

[120] Chunchui S, Weng N, Chang X, Feng L, Yao H, Wu N. Effect of allicin on THP-1, MT-2 and WISH cell apoptosis induced by vesicular stomatitis virus (VSV) and the molecular mechanism involved. Afr J Biotechnol 2011; 10(36): 7040-7.https://www.ajol.info/index.php/ajb/article/view/94708 [cited 28th November 2020].

[121] Zhao S, Jia Y, Zhang W, Mao Y, Teng K. Oral administration of *Allium sativum* extract protects against infectious bursal disease in chickens[J]. Front Agr Sci Eng 2015; 2(4): 318-326.

[122] Wang L, Jiao H, Zhao J, Wang X, Sun S, Lin H. Allicin alleviates reticuloendotheliosis virus-induced immunosuppression *via* ERK/mitogen-activated protein kinase pathway in specific pathogen-free chickens. Front Immunol. 2017; 8:1856.

[123] Josling P. Preventing the common cold with a garlic supplement: a double-blind, placebo-controlled survey. Adv Ther 2001; 18(4): 189-93. http://www.bravacorp.com/garlic%20and%20the%20common%20cold.pdf [cited 29th November 2020]. [http://dx.doi.org/10.1007/BF02850113] [PMID: 11697022]

[124] Andrianova IV, Sobenin IA, Sereda EV, Borodina LI, Studenikin MI. Effect of long-acting garlic tablets "allicor" on the incidence of acute respiratory viral infections in children. Ter Arkh 2003; 75(3): 53-6. [cited 29th November 2020]. [PMID: 12718222]

[125] Mäkelä MJ, Puhakka T, Ruuskanen O, *et al.* Viruses and bacteria in the etiology of the common cold. J Clin Microbiol 1998; 36(2): 539-42.https://www.ncbi.nlm.nih.gov/pmc/articles/PMC104573/ [cited 29th November 2020]. [http://dx.doi.org/10.1128/JCM.36.2.539-542.1998] [PMID: 9466772]

[126] Small LD, Bailey JH, Cavallito CJ. Alkyl thiolsulfinates. J Am Chem Soc. 1947 Jul;69(7):1710-3.

[127] Lubenets V, Vasylyuk S, Monka N, *et al.* Synthesis and antimicrobial properties of 4-acylaminobenzenethiosulfoacid S-esters. Saudi Pharm J 2017; 25(2): 266-74. [cited 29th November 2020]. [http://dx.doi.org/10.1016/j.jsps.2016.06.007] [PMID: 28344478]

[128] Sheppard JG, McAleer JP, Saralkar P, Geldenhuys WJ, Long TE. Allicin-inspired pyridyl disulfides as antimicrobial agents for multidrug-resistant *Staphylococcus aureus*. Eur J Med Chem 2018; 143:1185-1195.

[129] Qi F, Zhang C, Jiang S, *et al.* S-ethyl ethanethiosulfinate, a derivative of allicin, induces metacaspase-dependent apoptosis through ROS generation in Penicillium chrysogenum. Biosci Rep 2019; 39 (6): BSR20190167.

[130] Rablen PR, Perry-Freer NA. Perry-Freer NA. How the arrangement of alkyl substituents affects the stability of delocalized carbocations. The Journal of Organic Chemistry 2018; 83 (7): 4024-4033. [http://dx.doi.org/10.1021/acs.joc.8b00415]

[131] Luo DQ, Guo JH, Wang FJ, *et al.* Anti-fungal Efficacy of Polybutylcyanoacrylate Nanoparticles of Allicin and Comparison With Pure Allicin, Journal of Biomaterials Science, Polymer Edition 2009; 20(1): 21-31.

[132] Pirak T, Jangchud A, Jantawat P. Characterisation of physical, chemical and antimicrobial properties

of allicin–chitosan complexes. Int J Food Sci Technol 2012; 47: 1339-47. [cited 30th November 2020]. [http://dx.doi.org/10.1111/j.1365-2621.2012.02978.x]

[133] Jebali A, Hekmatimoghaddam S, Behzadi A, *et al.* Antimicrobial activity of nanocellulose conjugated with allicin and lysozyme. Cellulose 2013; 20: 2897-907. [cited 30th November 2020]. [http://dx.doi.org/10.1007/s10570-013-0084-3]

[134] Jafary R, Mehrizi MK, Hekmatimoghaddam SH, Jebali A. Antibacterial property of cellulose fabric finished by allicin-conjugated nanocellulose, The Journal of The Textile Institute 2015; 106:7, 683-689.

[135] Sharifi-Rad J, Hoseini Alfatemi S, Sharifi Rad M, Iriti M. Antimicrobial synergic effect of allicin and silver nanoparticles on skin infection caused by methicillin-resistant *Staphylococcus aureus* spp. Ann Med Health Sci Res 2014; 4(6): 863-868.

[136] Mirzaei F, Salouti M, Shapouri R. Effect of Allicin and Silver Nanoparticles on Skin Infections Due to *Staphylococcus aureus* in Mouse Model. J Adv Med Biomed Res 2015; 23(97): 94-102.http://zums.ac.ir/journal/article-1-3091-en.html [cited 30th November 2020].

[137] Thanka Rajan S, Karthika M, Balaji U, Muthappan A, Subramanian B. Functional finishing of medical fabrics using CeO_2/allicin nanocomposite for wound dressings. J Alloys Compd 2017; 695: 747-52. [cited 30th November 2020]. [http://dx.doi.org/10.1016/j.jallcom.2016.06.241]

[138] Soumya RS, Sherin S, Raghu KG, Abraham A. Allicin functionalized locust bean gum nanoparticles for improved therapeutic efficacy: An *in silico, in vitro* and *in vivo* approach. Int J Biol Macromol 2018; 109: 740-7. [cited 30th November 2020]. [http://dx.doi.org/10.1016/j.ijbiomac.2017.11.065] [PMID: 29155156]

[139] Roy T, Catlin NS, Garner DM, Cantino PD, Scheen AC, Lindqvist C. Evolutionary relationships within the lamioid tribe Synandreae (Lamiaceae) based on multiple low-copy nuclear loci. PeerJ 2016;4:e2220.

[140] De Martino L, De Feo V, Formisano C, Mignola E, Senatore F. Chemical composition and antimicrobial activity of the essential oils from three chemotypes of *Origanum vulgare* L. ssp. hirtum (Link) Ietswaart growing wild in Campania (Southern Italy). Molecules 2009; 14(8): 2735-46. [http://dx.doi.org/10.3390/molecules14082735] [PMID: 19701120]

[141] Jan S, Rashid M, Abd Allah EF, Ahmad P. Biological efficacy of essential oils and plant extracts of cultivated and wild ecotypes of *Origanum vulgare L.* BioMed Res Int 2020; 2020: 8751718. [cited 9th December 2020]. [http://dx.doi.org/10.1155/2020/8751718] [PMID: 32337282]

[142] Baser KHC. The Turkish Origanum series. In: Keszios SE, Ed. Oregano the genera Origanum and Lippia. London, New York: Taylor and Francis 2002; pp. 109-26.

[143] Brđanin S, Bogdanović N, Kolundžić M, *et al.* Antimicrobial activity of oregano (Origanum vulgare L.) and basil (Ocimum basilicum L.): Extracts. Advanced Technologies 2015;4(2): 5-10. https://core.ac.uk/download/pdf/237392863.pdf

[144] Andrews AC. Hyssop in the classical era. Classical Philosophy 1961; 56(4):230-248. https://www.journals.uchicago.edu/doi/10.1086/364619 [http://dx.doi.org/10.1086/364619]

[145] [Carvacrol] In IUPAC Standards Online (2017). Berlin, Boston: De Gruyter. https://db.degruyter.com/view/IUPAC/iupac.compound.10364

[146] Voelckel FC. Über die Zusammensetzung des Cascarill- und des Kümmelöls. Ann Chem Pharm 1840; 35: 306-9. [http://dx.doi.org/10.1002/jlac.18400350308]

[147] (1818-1860) the unknown chemist and his well-known reagent. Chem Educ 1984; 61(12): 1095-6. [cited 9th December 2020].

[http://dx.doi.org/10.1021/ed061p1095]

[148] Hixson AW, McKee RW. A study of the conditions essential for the commercial manufacture of carvacrol. Journal of Industrial & Engineering Chemistry 1918; 10(12): 982-992. [http://dx.doi.org/10.1021/ie50108a016]

[149] Suntres ZE, Coccimiglio J, Alipour M. The bioactivity and toxicological actions of carvacrol. Crit Rev Food Sci Nutr. 2015;55(3):304-18. [http://dx.doi.org/10.1080/10408398.2011.653458]

[150] Chavan PS, Tupe SG. Antifungal activity and mechanism of action of carvacrol and thymol against vineyard and wine spoilage yeasts. Food Control 2014; 46: 115-20. [cited 9th December 2020]. [http://dx.doi.org/10.1016/j.foodcont.2014.05.007]

[151] Chami N, Chami F, Bennis S, Trouillas J, Remmal A. Antifungal treatment with carvacrol and eugenol of oral candidiasis in immunosuppressed rats. Braz J Infect Dis 2004; 8(3): 217-26. [cited 9th December 2020]. [http://dx.doi.org/10.1590/S1413-86702004000300005] [PMID: 15476054]

[152] Mediouni S, Jablonski JA, Tsuda S. Oregano Oil and Its Principal Component, Carvacrol, Inhibit HIV-1 Fusion into Target Cells. Journal of Virology Jul 2020, 94 (15) e00147-20.

[153] Kumar A, Choudhir G, Shukla SK, *et al.* Identification of phytochemical inhibitors against main protease of COVID-19 using molecular modeling approaches [published online ahead of print, 2020 Jun 4]. J Biomol Struct Dyn 2020;1-11.

[154] Gilling DH, Kitajima M, Torrey JR, Bright KR. Antiviral efficacy and mechanisms of action of oregano essential oil and its primary component carvacrol against murine norovirus. J Appl Microbiol 2014; 116(5): 1149-63. [cited 9th December 2020]. [http://dx.doi.org/10.1111/jam.12453] [PMID: 24779581]

[155] Sharifi-Rad J, Salehi B, Schnitzler P, *et al.* Susceptibility of herpes simplex virus type 1 to monoterpenes thymol, carvacrol, p-cymene and essential oils of Sinapis arvensis L., Lallemantia royleana Benth. and Pulicaria vulgaris Gaertn. Cell Mol Biol (Noisy-le-grand) 2017;63(8):42-47.

[156] Magi G, Marini E, Facinelli B. Antimicrobial activity of essential oils and carvacrol, and synergy of carvacrol and erythromycin, against clinical, erythromycin-resistant Group A Streptococci. Front Microbiol. 2015; 6:165. [http://dx.doi.org/10.3389/fmicb.2015.00165]

[157] Du E, Gan L, Li Z, Wang W, Liu D, Guo Y. *In vitro* antibacterial activity of thymol and carvacrol and their effects on broiler chickens challenged with *Clostridium perfringens.* J Anim Sci Biotechnol 2015; 6: 58. [cited 9th December 2020]. [http://dx.doi.org/10.1186/s40104-015-0055-7] [PMID: 26705471]

[158] Tasdemir D, Kaiser M, Demirci B, Demirci F, Baser KHC. Antiprotozoal Activity of Turkish Origanum onites Essential Oil and Its Components. Molecules 2019;24(23):4421.

[159] Youssefi MR, Moghaddas E, Tabari MA, *et al. In vitro* and *in vivo* Effectiveness of Carvacrol, Thymol and Linalool against Leishmania infantum. Molecules 2019;24(11):2072.

[160] Tanghort M, Chefchaou H, Mzabi A, *et al.* Oocysticidal Effect of Essential Oils (EOs) and their Major Components on *Cryptosporidium baileyi* and *Cryptosporidium galli.* Int J Poult Sci 2019; 18: 475-82.https://scialert.net/fulltext/?doi=ijps.2019.475.482 [cited on 9th December 2020]. [http://dx.doi.org/10.3923/ijps.2019.475.482]

[161] Echeverrigaray S, Zacaria J, Beltrão R. Nematicidal activity of monoterpenoids against the root-knot nematode *Meloidogyne incognita.* Phytopathology. 2010;100(2):199-203.

[162] Souza EL, Stamford MTLM, Lima EO, Filho JMB, Marques MOM. Interference of heating on the antimicrobial activity and chemical composition of *Origanum vulgare* L. (*Lamiaceae*) essential oil. Food Sci Technol (Campinas) 2008; 28(2): 418-22. [cited 9th December 2020]. [http://dx.doi.org/10.1590/S0101-20612008000200023]

[163] Guevara L, Antolinos V, Palop A, Periago PM. Impact of moderate heat, carvacrol and thymol treatments on the viability, injury and stress response of *Listeria monocytogenes*. BioMed Res Int 2015; 2015: 548930. [cited 9th December 2020].
[http://dx.doi.org/10.1155/2015/548930] [PMID: 26539510]

[164] Lambert RJW, Skandamis PN, Coote PJ, Nychas G-JE. A study of the minimum inhibitory concentration and mode of action of oregano essential oil, thymol and carvacrol. J Appl Microbiol 2001; 91(3): 453-62. [cited 9th December 2020].
[http://dx.doi.org/10.1046/j.1365-2672.2001.01428.x] [PMID: 11556910]

[165] Yildiz ZI, Celebioglu A, Kilic ME, *et al.* Fast-dissolving carvacrol/cyclodextrin inclusion complex electrospun fibers with enhanced thermal stability, water solubility, and antioxidant activity. J Mater Sci 2018; 53: 15837-49. [cited 9th December 2020].
[http://dx.doi.org/10.1007/s10853-018-2750-1]

[166] Schroeder J, Vollmer H. The excretion of thymol, carvacrol, eugenol and guaiacol and the distribution of these substances in the organism. Arch Exp Path Pharmacol 1932; 168: 331-53.

[167] Opdyke DL. Monographs on fragrance raw materials. Food Cosmet Toxicol 1979; 17(Special Issue V.): 695-923.
[PMID: 540894]

[168] Austgulen L-T, Solheim E, Scheline RR. Metabolism in rats of *p*-cymene derivatives: carvacrol and thymol. Pharmacol Toxicol 1987; 61(2): 98-102. [cited 9th November 2020].
[http://dx.doi.org/10.1111/j.1600-0773.1987.tb01783.x] [PMID: 2959918]

[169] Lu Y, Wu C. Reduction of Salmonella enterica contamination on grape tomatoes by washing with thyme oil, thymol, and carvacrol as compared with chlorine treatment. J Food Prot 2010; 73(12): 2270-5. [cited 9th December 2020].
[http://dx.doi.org/10.4315/0362-028X-73.12.2270] [PMID: 21219747]

[170] Gong J, Yin F, Hou Y, Yin Y. Review: Chinese herbs as alternatives to antibiotics in feed for swine and poultry production: Potential and challenges in application. Can J Anim Sci 2013; 94(2): 223-41. [cited 9th December 2020].
[http://dx.doi.org/10.4141/cjas2013-144]

[171] Zhai H, Liu H, Wang S, Wu J, Kluenter A-M. Potential of essential oils for poultry and pigs. Anim Nutr 2018; 4(2): 179-86. [cited 9th December 2020].
[http://dx.doi.org/10.1016/j.aninu.2018.01.005] [PMID: 30140757]

[172] Kirchhelle C. Pharming animals: a global history of antibiotics in food production (1935–2017). Palgrave Commun 2018; 4: 96. [cited 9th December 2020].
[http://dx.doi.org/10.1057/s41599-018-0152-2]

[173] Khan ST, Khan M, Ahmad J, *et al.* Thymol and carvacrol induce autolysis, stress, growth inhibition and reduce the biofilm formation by Streptococcus mutans. AMB Express 2017;7(1):49.

[174] Nosrat A, Bolhari B, Sharifian MR, Aligholi M, Mortazavi MS. The effect of Carvacrol on *Enterococcus faecalis* as a final irrigant. Iran Endod J 2009; 4(3): 96-100.https://www.ncbi.nlm.nih.gov/pmc/articles/PMC3758867/ [cited 9th December 2020].
[PMID: 24003329]

[175] Oke F, Aslim B, Ozturk S, Altundag S. Essential oil composition, antimicrobial and antioxidant activities of *Satureja cuneifolia* Ten. Food Chem 2009; 112(4): 874-9. [cited 9th December 2020].
[http://dx.doi.org/10.1016/j.foodchem.2008.06.061]

[176] Keawchaoon L, Yoksan R. Preparation, characterization and *in vitro* release study of carvacrol-loaded chitosan nanoparticles. Colloids Surf B Biointerfaces 2011; 84(1): 163-71. [cited 9th December 2020].
[http://dx.doi.org/10.1016/j.colsurfb.2010.12.031] [PMID: 21296562]

[177] Windiasti G, Feng J, Lina Ma L, *et al.* Investigating the synergistic antimicrobial effect of carvacrol and zinc oxide nanoparticles against *Campylobacter jejuni*. Food Control 2019; 96: 39-46. [cited 9th

December 2020].
[http://dx.doi.org/10.1016/j.foodcont.2018.08.028]

[178] He J, Huang S, Sun X, *et al.* Carvacrol Loaded Solid Lipid Nanoparticles of Propylene Glycol Monopalmitate and Glyceryl Monostearate: Preparation, Characterization, and Synergistic Antimicrobial Activity. Nanomaterials (Basel) 2019; 9(8): 1162. [cited 9th December 2020]. [http://dx.doi.org/10.3390/nano9081162] [PMID: 31416170]

[179] Niza E, Božik M, Bravo I, *et al.* PEI-coated PLA nanoparticles to enhance the antimicrobial activity of carvacrol. Food Chem 2020; 328: 127131. [cited 9th December 2020]. [http://dx.doi.org/10.1016/j.foodchem.2020.127131] [PMID: 32485586]

[180] Mauriello E, Ferrari G, Donsì F. Effect of formulation on properties, stability, carvacrol release and antimicrobial activity of carvacrol emulsions. Colloids Surf B Biointerfaces 2021; 197: 111424. [cited 9th December 2020]. [http://dx.doi.org/10.1016/j.colsurfb.2020.111424] [PMID: 33099148]

[181] Ultee A, Bennik MH, Moezelaar R. The phenolic hydroxyl group of carvacrol is essential for action against the food-borne pathogen Bacillus cereus. Appl Environ Microbiol 2002;68(4):1561-1568.

[182] Ben Arfa A, Combes S, Preziosi-Belloy L, Gontard N, Chalier P. Antimicrobial activity of carvacrol related to its chemical structure. Lett Appl Microbiol 2006; 43(2): 149-54. [cited 11th December 2020]. [http://dx.doi.org/10.1111/j.1472-765X.2006.01938.x] [PMID: 16869897]

[183] Reiner GN, Labuckas DO, García DA, García DA. Lipophilicity of some GABAergic phenols and related compounds determined by HPLC and partition coefficients in different systems. J Pharm Biomed Anal 2009; 49(3): 686-91. [cited 28th February 2021]. [http://dx.doi.org/10.1016/j.jpba.2008.12.040] [PMID: 19188039]

[184] Reiner GN, Perillo MA, García DA. Effects of propofol and other GABAergic phenols on membrane molecular organization. Colloids Surf B Biointerfaces 2013; 101: 61-7. [cited 28th February 2021]. [http://dx.doi.org/10.1016/j.colsurfb.2012.06.004] [PMID: 22796773]

[185] Miguel V, Villarreal MA, García DA. Effects of gabergic phenols on the dynamic and structure of lipid bilayers: A molecular dynamic simulation approach. PLoS One 2019; 14(6): e0218042. [cited 28th February 2021]. [http://dx.doi.org/10.1371/journal.pone.0218042] [PMID: 31237897]

[186] Churklam W, Chaturongakul S, Ngamwongsatit B, Aunpad R. The mechanisms of action of carvacrol and its synergism with nisin against *Listeria monocytogenes* on sliced bologna sausage. Food Control 2020; 108: 106864. [cited 11th December 2020]. [http://dx.doi.org/10.1016/j.foodcont.2019.106864]

[187] Gill AO, Holley RA. Disruption of *Escherichia coli*, *Listeria monocytogenes* and *Lactobacillus sakei* cellular membranes by plant oil aromatics. Int J Food Microbiol. 2006; 108(1): 1-9.

[188] Gill AO, Holley RA. Inhibition of membrane bound ATPases of *Escherichia coli* and *Listeria monocytogenes* by plant oil aromatics. International Journal of Food Microbiology 2006; 111(2): 170:174.

[189] Mith H, Clinquart A, Zhiri A, Daube G, Delcenserie V. The impact of oregano (Origanum heracleoticum) essential oil and carvacrol on virulence gene transcription by *Escherichia coli* O157: H7. FEMS Microbiol Lett 2015; 362(1): 1-7.

[190] Wagle BR, Upadhyay A, Upadhyaya I, *et al.* Trans-Cinnamaldehyde, Eugenol and Carvacrol Reduce *Campylobacter jejuni* Biofilms and Modulate Expression of Select Genes and Proteins. Frontiers in Microbiology 2019; 10:1837.

[191] Myszka K, Schmidt MT, Majcher M, Juzwa W, Olkowicz M, Czaczyk K. Inhibition of quorum sensing-related biofilm of *Pseudomonas fluorescens* KM121 by *Thymus vulgare* essential oil and its major bioactive compounds. Int Biodeterior Biodegradation 2016; 114: 252-9. [cited 15th December 2020].

[http://dx.doi.org/10.1016/j.ibiod.2016.07.006]

[192] Shapira R, Mimran E. Isolation and characterization of *Escherichia coli* mutants exhibiting altered response to thymol. Microb Drug Resist 2007; 13: 157–165.

[193] Nostro A, Cellini L, Zimbalatti V, *et al.* Enhanced activity of carvacrol against biofilm of *Staphylococcus aureus* and *Staphylococcus epidermidis* in an acidic environment. APMIS. 2012;120(12):967-73.

[194] Tapia-Rodriguez MR, Hernandez-Mendoza A, Gonzalez-Aguilar GA, Martinez-Tellez MA, Miranda Martins C, Ayala-Zavala FJ. Carvacrol as potential quorum sensing inhibitor of *Pseudomonas aeruginosa* and biofilm production on stainless steel surfaces. Food Control 2017; 75: 255-61. [cited 15th December 2020].
[http://dx.doi.org/10.1016/j.foodcont.2016.12.014]

[195] Burt SA, Ojo-Fakunle VTA, Woertman J, Veldhuizen EJA. The natural antimicrobial carvacrol inhibits quorum sensing in *Chromobacterium violaceum* and reduces bacterial biofilm formation at sub-lethal concentrations. PLoS One 2014; 9(4): e93414. [cited 15th December 2020].
[http://dx.doi.org/10.1371/journal.pone.0093414] [PMID: 24691035]

[196] Trevisan DAC, da Silva AF, Negri M, *et al.* Antibacterial and antibiofilm activity of carvacrol against *Salmonella enterica* serotype Typhimurium. Braz J Pharm Sci 2018; 54(1): e17229. [cited 15th December 2020].
[http://dx.doi.org/10.1590/s2175-97902018000117229]

[197] Čabarkapa IC, Škrinjar MM, Lević JD, *et al.* . Influence of carvacrol and thymol on initial cell attachment and biofilm of *Candida albicans* . Food and Feed Research 2015; 42(1):23-30.

[198] Kumari P, Mishra R, Arora N, *et al.* Antifungal and anti-biofilm activity of essential oil active components against *Cryptococcus neoformans* and *Cryptococcus laurentii*. Front Microbiol. 2017; 8: 2161.

[199] Ahmad A, Khan A, Akhtar F, *et al.* Fungicidal activity of thymol and carvacrol by disrupting ergosterol biosynthesis and membrane integrity against Candida. Eur J Clin Microbiol Infect Dis. 2011;30(1):41-50.
[http://dx.doi.org/10.1007/s10096-010-1050-8]

[200] Nóbrega RO, Teixeira AP, Oliveira WA, Lima EO, Lima IO. Investigation of the antifungal activity of carvacrol against strains of *Cryptococcus neoformans* . Pharm Biol 2016; 54(11): 2591-6.
[http://dx.doi.org/10.3109/13880209.2016.1172319] [PMID: 27225838]

[201] Albuquerque P, Casadevall A. Quorum sensing in fungi--a review. Med Mycol 2012; 50(4): 337-45. [cited 15th December 2020].
[http://dx.doi.org/10.3109/13693786.2011.652201] [PMID: 22268493]

[202] Karuppannasamy S, Narayanan K, Pillai CN. Reactions of phenols and alcohols over thoria: Mechanism of ether formation. J Catal 1980; 66(2): 281-9. [cited 15th December 2020].
[http://dx.doi.org/10.1016/0021-9517(80)90032-9]

[203] Stone NR, Bicanic T, Salim R, Hope W. Liposomal amphotericin B (AmBisome(®): a review of the pharmacokinetics, pharmacodynamics, clinical experience and future directions. Drugs 2016; 76(4): 485-500.

[204] Wang LH, Wang MS, Zeng XA, Zhang ZH, Gong DM, Huang YB. Membrane destruction and DNA binding of *Staphylococcus aureus* cells induced by carvacrol and its combined effect with a pulsed electric field. J Agric Food Chem. 2016; 64(32): 6355-63.

[205] Siroli L, Braschi G, de Jong A, Kok J, Patrignani F, Lanciotti R. Transcriptomic approach and membrane fatty acid analysis to study the response mechanisms of *Escherichia coli* to thyme essential oil, carvacrol, 2-(E)-hexanal and citral exposure. J Appl Microbiol. 2018;125(5):1308-1320.

[206] Berdejo D, Chueca B, Pagán E, *et al.* Sub-Inhibitory Doses of Individual Constituents of Essential Oils Can Select for *Staphylococcus aureus* Resistant Mutants. Molecules 2019;24(1):170.

[207] Haiko J, Westerlund-Wikström B. The role of the bacterial flagellum in adhesion and virulence. Biology (Basel) 2013;2(4):1242-1267. [http://dx.doi.org/10.3390/biology2041242]

[208] Clyne M, Ocroinin T, Suerbaum S, Josenhans C, Drumm B. Adherence of isogenic flagellum-negative mutants of *Helicobacter pylori* and *Helicobacter mustelae* to human and ferret gastric epithelial cells. Infect Immun 2000; 68: 4335–4339.

[209] Kalmakoff M, Lanthier P, Tremblay T-L, *et al.* Proteomic analysis of *Campylobacter jejuni* 11168 biofilms reveals a role for the motility complex in biofilm formation. Journal of Bacteriology 2006; 188 (12) 4312-4320.

[210] Kim JS, Park C, Kim YJ. Role of flgA for Flagellar Biosynthesis and Biofilm Formation of *Campylobacter jejuni* NCTC11168. J Microbiol Biotechnol 2015; 25(11): 1871-9. [cited 15th December 2020]. [http://dx.doi.org/10.4014/jmb.1504.04080] [PMID: 26215271]

[211] Rao A, Zhang Y, Muend S, Rao R. Mechanism of Antifungal Activity of Terpenoid Phenols Resembles Calcium Stress and Inhibition of the TOR Pathway. Antimicrobial Agents and Chemotherapy Nov 2010;54 (12): 5062-5069. [http://dx.doi.org/10.1128/AAC.01050-10]

[212] Roelants FM, Chauhan N, Muir A, *et al.* TOR complex 2-regulated protein kinase Ypk1 controls sterol distribution by inhibiting StARkin domain-containing proteins located at plasma membrane-endoplasmic reticulum contact sites. Mol Biol Cell 2018; 29(17):2128-2136.

[213] Chaillot J, Tebbji F, Remmal A, *et al.* The Monoterpene Carvacrol Generates Endoplasmic Reticulum Stress in the Pathogenic Fungus *Candida albicans* . Antimicrob Agents Chemother 2015;59(8):4584-4592.

[214] Kamalabadi M, Astani A, Nemati F. Anti-viral Effect and Mechanism of Carvacrol on Herpes Simplex Virus Type 1. IJML. 2018; 5 (2) :113-122. http://ijml.ssu.ac.ir/article-1-196-en.html

[215] Kieff E, Hoyer B, Bachenheimer S, Roizman B. Genetic relatedness of type 1 and type 2 herpes simplex viruses. J Virol 1972;9(5):738-745.

[216] Wang L, Wang D, Wu X, Xu R, Li Y. Antiviral mechanism of carvacrol on HSV-2 infectivity through inhibition of RIP3-mediated programmed cell necrosis pathway and ubiquitin-proteasome system in BSC-1 cells. BMC Infect Dis 2020; 20(1): 832. [cited 16th December 2020]. [http://dx.doi.org/10.1186/s12879-020-05556-9] [PMID: 33176697]

[217] Joshi RS, Jagdale SS, Bansode SB, *et al.* Discovery of potential multi-target-directed ligands by targeting host-specific SARS-CoV-2 structurally conserved main protease [published online ahead of print, 2020 May 5]. J Biomol Struct Dyn 2020;1-16.

[218] Kortman GA, Roelofs RW, Swinkels DW, de Jonge MI, Burt SA, Tjalsma H. Iron-induced virulence of Salmonella enterica serovar typhimurium at the intestinal epithelial interface can be suppressed by carvacrol. Antimicrob Agents Chemother 2014;58(3):1664-1670.

[219] Marchese A, Arciola CR, Coppo E, *et al.* The natural plant compound carvacrol as an antimicrobial and anti-biofilm agent: mechanisms, synergies and bio-inspired anti-infective materials. Biofouling 2018;34(6):630-656. [http://dx.doi.org/10.1080/08927014.2018.1480756]

[220] Espina L, Pagán R, López D, García-Gonzalo D. Individual Constituents from Essential Oils Inhibit Biofilm Mass Production by Multi-Drug Resistant *Staphylococcus aureus*. Molecules. 2015;20(6):11357-11372.

[221] Al-Ani I, Zimmermann S, Reichling J, Wink M. Pharmacological synergism of bee venom and melittin with antibiotics and plant secondary metabolites against multi-drug resistant microbial pathogens. Phytomedicine 2015;22(2):245-55. [http://dx.doi.org/10.1016/j.phymed.2014.11.019]

[222] Souza EL, Oliveira CE, Stamford TL, Conceição ML, Neto NJ. Influence of carvacrol and thymol on the physiological attributes, enterotoxin production and surface characteristics of *Staphylococcus aureus* strains isolated from foods. Braz J Microbiol. 2013;44(1):29-35.

[223] Mooyottu S, Kollanoor-Johny A, Flock G, *et al.* Carvacrol and trans-cinnamaldehyde reduce Clostridium difficile toxin production and cytotoxicity *in vitro*. Int J Mol Sci. 2014;15(3):4415-4430.

[224] Upadhyay A, Johny AK, Amalaradjou MA, Ananda Baskaran S, Kim KS, Venkitanarayanan K. Plant-derived antimicrobials reduce *Listeria monocytogenes* virulence factors *in vitro*, and down-regulate expression of virulence genes. Int J Food Microbiol 15;157(1):88-94.

[225] Upadhyay A, Mooyottu S, Yin H, Nair MS, Bhattaram V, Venkitanarayanan K. Inhibiting Microbial Toxins Using Plant-Derived Compounds and Plant Extracts. Medicines (Basel) 2015;2(3):186-211. [http://dx.doi.org/10.3390/medicines2030186]

[226] Kidsley AK, Abraham S, Bell JM, *et al.* Antimicrobial Susceptibility of *Escherichia coli* and Salmonella spp. Isolates From Healthy Pigs in Australia: Results of a Pilot National Survey. Front Microbiol 2018; 9:1207.

[227] Oliveira L, Langoni H, Hulland C, Ruegg PL. Minimum inhibitory concentrations of *Staphylococcus aureus* recovered from clinical and subclinical cases of bovine mastitis. J Dairy Sci 2012; 95(4): 1913-20. [cited 18th December].
[http://dx.doi.org/10.3168/jds.2011-4938] [PMID: 22459838]

[228] Cirino IC, Menezes-Silva SM, Silva HT, de Souza EL, Siqueira-Júnior JP. The Essential Oil from *Origanum vulgare* L. and Its Individual Constituents Carvacrol and Thymol Enhance the Effect of Tetracycline against *Staphylococcus aureus* . Chemotherapy. 2014;60(5-6):290-3.

[229] Zanini SF, Silva-Angulo AB, Rosenthal A, Rodrigo D, Martínez A. Effect of citral and carvacrol on the susceptibility of *Listeria monocytogenes* and *Listeria innocua* to antibiotics. Lett Appl Microbiol. 2014; 58(5): 486-92.

[230] Zuzarte M, Vale-Silva L, Gonçalves MJ, *et al.* Antifungal activity of phenolic-rich *Lavandula multifida* L. essential oil. Eur J Clin Microbiol Infect Dis. 2012;31(7):1359-66.

[231] Vale-Silva L, Silva MJ, Oliveira D, *et al.* Correlation of the chemical composition of essential oils from Origanum vulgare subsp. virens with their *in vitro* activity against pathogenic yeasts and filamentous fungi. J Med Microbiol. 2012; 61(2):252-260.

[232] Ahmad A, Khan A, Manzoor N. Reversal of efflux mediated antifungal resistance underlies synergistic activity of two monoterpenes with fluconazole. Eur J Pharm Sci 2013; 48(1-2): 80-6. [cited 18th December 2020].
[http://dx.doi.org/10.1016/j.ejps.2012.09.016] [PMID: 23111348]

[233] Abbaszadeh S, Sharifzadeh A, Shokri H, Khosravi AR, Abbaszadeh A. Antifungal efficacy of thymol, carvacrol, eugenol and menthol as alternative agents to control the growth of food-relevant fungi. J Mycol Med 2014; 24(2):e51-6.

[234] Mahboubi M. The anti-dermatophyte activity of *Zataria multiflora* essential oils. J Mycol Med 2017;27(2):232-237.

[235] Jesus FP, Ferreiro L, Bizzi KS, *et al. In vitro* activity of carvacrol and thymol combined with antifungals or antibacterials against *Pythium insidiosum*. J Mycol Med. 2015; 25(2):e89-93.

[236] Liu Q, Qiao K, Zhang S. Potential of small molecule carvacrol in management of vegetable diseases. Molecules 2019; 24: 1932.

[237] Numpaque MA, Ovieda LA, Gil JH, García CM, Durango DL. Thymol and carvacrol: biotransformation and antifungal activity against the plant pathogenic fungi *Colletotrichum acutatum* and *Botryodiplodia theobromae.* Trop Plant Pathol 2011; 36(1): 3-13. [cited 18th December 2020].
[http://dx.doi.org/10.1590/S1982-56762011000100001]

[238] Hou H, Zhang X, Zhao T, Zhou L. Effects of *Origanum vulgare* essential oil and its two main

components, carvacrol and thymol, on the plant pathogen *Botrytis cinerea.* PeerJ 2020; 8: e9626. [cited 18th December 2020].
[http://dx.doi.org/10.7717/peerj.9626] [PMID: 32864206]

[239] Zhou D, Wang Z, Li M, Xing M, Xian T, Tu K. Carvacrol and eugenol effectively inhibit Rhizopus stolonifer and control postharvest soft rot decay in peaches. J Appl Microbiol 2018;124(1):166-178.

[240] Chami N, Chami F, Bennis S, Trouillas J, Remmal A. Antifungal treatment with carvacrol and eugenol of oral candidiasis in immunosuppressed rats. Braz J Infect Dis. 2004;8(3):217-26.
[http://dx.doi.org/10.1590/S1413-86702004000300005]

[241] Silva ARST, Scher R, Santos FV, *et al.* Leishmanicidal Activity and Structure-Activity Relationships of Essential Oil Constituents. Molecules. 2017;22(5):815.
[http://dx.doi.org/10.3390/molecules22050815]

[242] Oka Y, Nacar S, Eli Putievsky E, Ravid U, Yaniv Z, Spiegel Y. Nematicidal Activity of Essential Oils and Their Components Against the Root-Knot Nematode. Phytopathology 2000; 90(7):710-715.
[http://dx.doi.org/10.1094/PHYTO.2000.90.7.710]

[243] Pilau MR, Alves SH, Weiblen R, Arenhart S, Cueto AP, Lovato LT. Antiviral activity of the *Lippia graveolen*s (Mexican oregano) essential oil and its main compound carvacrol against human and animal viruses. Braz J Microbiol 2011; 42(4): 1616-24. [cited 18th December 2020].
[http://dx.doi.org/10.1590/S1517-83822011000400049] [PMID: 24031796]

[244] Ma L, Yao L. Antiviral Effects of Plant-Derived Essential Oils and Their Components: An Updated Review. Molecules 2020;25(11):2627.

[245] Mathela CS, Singh KK, Gupta VK. Synthesis and *in vitro* antibacterial activity of thymol and carvacrol derivatives. Acta Pol Pharm 2010; 67(4): 375-80. https://www.ptfarm.pl/pub/File/Acta_Poloniae/2010/4/375.pdf [cited 18th December 2020].
[PMID: 20635533]

[246] Walsh DJ, Livinghouse T, Goeres DM, Mettler M, Stewart PS. Antimicrobial Activity of Naturally Occurring Phenols and Derivatives Against Biofilm and Planktonic Bacteria. Front Chem. 2019; 7:653.
[http://dx.doi.org/10.3389/fchem.2019.00653]

[247] Cacciatore I, Di Giulio M, Fornasari E, *et al.* Carvacrol codrugs: a new approach in the antimicrobial plan. PLoS One 2015; 10(4): e0120937. [cited 18th December 2020].
[http://dx.doi.org/10.1371/journal.pone.0120937] [PMID: 25859852]

[248] Marinelli L, Fornasari E, Eusepi P, *et al.* Carvacrol prodrugs as novel antimicrobial agents. Eur J Med Chem 2019; 178: 515-29. [cited 18th December 2020].
[http://dx.doi.org/10.1016/j.ejmech.2019.05.093] [PMID: 31207463]

[249] Xavier FJ, Rodrigues KA, de Oliveira RG, *et al.* Synthesis and *in vitro* Anti Leishmania amazonensis Biological Screening of Morita-Baylis-Hillman Adducts Prepared from Eugenol, Thymol and Carvacrol. Molecules. 2016;21(11):1483.

[250] de Moraes J, Carvalho AAL, Nakano E, *et al.* Anthelmintic activity of carvacryl acetate against *Schistosoma mansoni* . Parasitol Res 2013; 112(2): 603-10. [cited 18th December 2020].
[http://dx.doi.org/10.1007/s00436-012-3172-7] [PMID: 23086444]

[251] Andre WP, Ribeiro WL, Cavalcante GS, *et al.* Comparative efficacy and toxic effects of carvacryl acetate and carvacrol on sheep gastrointestinal nematodes and mice. Vet Parasitol. 2016; 218:52-8.
[http://dx.doi.org/10.1016/j.vetpar.2016.01.001]

[252] Martínez-Sanz M, Bilbao-Sainz C, Du WX, *et al.* Antimicrobial Poly(lactic acid)-Based Nanofibres Developed by Solution Blow Spinning. J Nanosci Nanotechnol. 2015;15(1):616-27.

[253] Iannitelli A, Grande R, Di Stefano A, *et al.* Potential antibacterial activity of carvacrol-loaded poly(DL-lactide-co-glycolide) (PLGA) nanoparticles against microbial biofilm. Int J Mol Sci 2011;12(8):5039-5051.

[254] Landis RF, Gupta A, Lee YW, *et al.* Cross-Linked Polymer-Stabilized Nanocomposites for the Treatment of Bacterial Biofilms. ACS Nano 2017;11(1):946-952. [http://dx.doi.org/10.1021/acsnano.6b07537]

[255] Shakeri F, Shakeri S, Hojjatoleslami M. Preparation and characterization of carvacrol loaded polyhydroxybutyrate nanoparticles by nanoprecipitation and dialysis methods. J Food Sci. 2014;79(4): N697-705.

[256] Rao SQ, Xu GW, Zeng HW, *et al.* Physicochemical and antibacterial properties of fabricated ovalbumin-carvacrol gel nanoparticles. Food Funct. 2020;11(6):5133-5141.

[257] Tenci M, Rossi S, Aguzzi C, *et al.* Carvacrol/clay hybrids loaded into *in situ* gelling films. Int J Pharm. 2017; 531(2): 676-688.

[258] Castro DO, Tabary N, Martel B, Gandini A, Belgacem N, Bras J. Effect of different carboxylic acids in cyclodextrin functionalization of cellulose nanocrystals for prolonged release of carvacrol. Mater Sci Eng C 2016; 69: 1018-25. [cited 18th December 2020]. [http://dx.doi.org/10.1016/j.msec.2016.08.014] [PMID: 27612798]

[259] Glaive A-S, Modjinou T, Versace D-L. Design of antibacterial and sustainable antioxidant networks based on plant phenolic derivatives used as delivery system of carvacrol or tannic acid. ACS Sustain Chem& Eng 2017; 5(3): 2320-9. [cited 18th December 2020]. [http://dx.doi.org/10.1021/acssuschemeng.6b02655]

[260] Bernardos A, Marina T, Žáček P, *et al.* Antifungal effect of essential oil components against *Aspergillus niger* when loaded into silica mesoporous supports. J Sci Food Agric. 2015;95(14):2824-31.

[261] Gharbi A, Legigan T, Humblot V, Papot S, Berjeaud JM. Surface functionalization by covalent immobilization of an innovative carvacrol derivative to avoid fungal biofilm formation [published correction appears in AMB Express. 2015 Dec;5(1):141.

[262] Weibson APP, Paiva JR Jr, Cavalcante GS, *et al.* Chitosan Nanoparticles Loaded with Carvacrol and Carvacryl Acetate for Improved Anthelmintic Activity. J Braz Chem Soc 2020; 31(8): 1614-22. [cited 18th December 2020]. [http://dx.doi.org/10.21577/0103-5053.20200047]

[263] Chen F, Shi Z, Neoh KG, Kang ET. Antioxidant and antibacterial activities of eugenol and carvacrol-grafted chitosan nanoparticles. Biotechnol Bioeng. 2009;104(1):30-9. [http://dx.doi.org/10.1002/bit.22363]

[264] Valcourt C, Saulnier P, Umerska A, *et al.* Synergistic interactions between doxycycline and terpenic components of essential oils encapsulated within lipid nanocapsules against gram negative bacteria. Int J Pharm. 2016;498(1-2):23-31. [http://dx.doi.org/10.1016/j.ijpharm.2015.11.042]

[265] Engel JB, Heckler C, Tondo EC, Daroit DJ, da Silva Malheiros P. Antimicrobial activity of free and liposome-encapsulated thymol and carvacrol against Salmonella and *Staphylococcus aureus* adhered to stainless steel. Int J Food Microbiol. 2017; 252:18-23.

[266] Zhong H, Chan G, Hu Y, Hu H, Ouyang DA. Comprehensive map of fda-approved pharmaceutical products. Pharmaceutics. 2018; 10(4): 263.

[267] Mohs RC, Greig NH. Drug discovery and development: Role of basic biological research. Alzheimers Dement (NY) 2017; 3(4): 651-657.

[268] Lei J, Sun L, Huang S, *et al.* The antimicrobial peptides and their potential clinical applications. Am J Transl Res 2019; 11(7): 3919-31. [PMID: 31396309]

[269] Jackson N, Czaplewski L, Piddock LJV. Discovery and development of new antibacterial drugs: learning from experience? J Antimicrob Chemother 2018; 73(6): 1452-9. [cited 15th January 2021].

[http://dx.doi.org/10.1093/jac/dky019] [PMID: 29438542]

[270] de Castro DO, Tabary N, Martel B, *et al.* Controlled release of carvacrol and curcumin: bio-based food packaging by synergism action of TEMPO-oxidized cellulose nanocrystals and cyclodextrin. Cellulose 2018; 25; 1249–1263.

[271] Moniruzzaman M, Min T. Curcumin, curcumin nanoparticles and curcumin nanospheres: a review on their pharmacodynamics based on monogastric farm animal, poultry and fish nutrition. Pharmaceutics 2020; 12(5): 447.

CHAPTER 2

Plant Phenolics as an Alternative Source of Antimicrobial Compounds

Inamullah Hakeem Said[1,*] and **Nikolai Kuhnert**[1,*]

[1] *Department of life sciences and Chemistry, Jacobs University Bremen, 28759 Bremen, Germany*

Abstract: The use and search for new medicines and dietary supplements derived from plants have enhanced in the modern era. Plants are rich in a wide variety of secondary metabolites, such as tannins, terpenoids, alkaloids, and flavonoids, which have been found *in vitro* to have antimicrobial properties. Polyphenols are natural compounds characterized by a high structural variety, and their existence in plants makes them essential components. Increasingly, resistant bacteria require the continuous need for new and effective antibiotics. This class of natural products is becoming the target of anti-infective research, and many groups have identified that phenolic compounds are possessing broad-spectrum antibacterial and antiviral activity. Owing to interest in their biological activities, both the chemical structure of the phenolic moiety and any attached chemical groups define whether the polyphenol is bioactive or not. Compared to other phenolics, flavonoids class have been abundantly used in anti-infective research.

This chapter summarizes the application of polyphenol tested by various groups against infectious diseases caused by bacteria and viruses as pathogens. The reported MIC values are presented in a concise table, which is conflicting among different groups, possibly due to assay parameters and strain variation. However, it is shown that phenolic compounds have great potentials, which requires future research for the development of novel antimicrobial or antiviral agents or aid as a synergistic agent in combination with conventional anti-infective drugs.

Keywords: Antibacterial, Antiviral, Plants, Polyphenols, Secondary metabolites.

INTRODUCTION

According to the European Union estimation in 2007, approximately 25,000 patients per annum die due to infection with major types of drug-resistant bacteria, which are responsible for bloodstream infection [1].

* **Corresponding authors Inamullah Hakeem Said & Nikolai Kuhnert:** Department of life sciences and Chemistry, Jacobs University Bremen, 28759 Bremen, Germany; E-mails: i.hakeemsaid@jacobs-university.de and n.kuhnert@jacobs-university.de

Ferid Murad, Atta-ur-Rahman, Ka Bian (Eds.)

Increasingly, resistant bacteria require a continuous need for new and effective antibiotics. However, in the last two-three decades, only two new classes of antimicrobials were launched in the market. Many drug developers have left the field. The medical interventions in the 21st century extended and improved our lives, such as anti-cancer drugs, cardiac surgery, transplantation, bone marrow transplantation and joint replacements. All mentioned interventions require strict control of infection. Although the current research could routinely add new medicines and therapies to address numerous other diseases, unfortunately, our grip on infection is loosening.

The agents (bacteria, viruses, fungi, and parasites) that cause infectious disease are continually trying to avoid and by-pass the drugs that are essential for combatting infection. In the past decades, scientists have countered the loss of potency of antibiotics resulting from resistance to the discovery and development of new ones. Over the past half-century, the strategy of introducing new antibiotics to the market to replace older ones, which lost their effectiveness has proven to be highly successful. Unfortunately, this state of equilibrium has now been shifted. Microbes have developed multiple drug resistance mechanisms, and no new antibiotic has been discovered [2].

Structural modification of existing antimicrobials to which bacteria have developed resistance such as the azoles [3], the non-nucleoside reverse transcriptase inhibitors [4], ß-lactams and quinolones [5] were effective means of extending the lifespan. However, with the selection of chemotherapeutics these days, the researchers are finding alternative ways to find new antimicrobials and do not follow the track of parent structure alterations. One of the recent development is to focus on different target sites to those in current use in finding novel antibiotics [6, 7].

In the past, natural products were also the major promising sources of chemical diversity for starting materials of drug discovery [8], for example, the penicillins, the tetracyclines and the glycopeptides between 1940 and 1955. In almost all therapeutic areas, many natural products or synthetically modified natural product derivatives are successfully produced for clinical use to treat various human diseases [9].

It is an ancient idea to find the healing powers in plants. Both in eastern and western culture, plants have been used for food and medicinal purposes for many centuries. In general, chemical extracts of plants are tested for a desirable activity, *i.e.*, antimicrobial, anticancer and anti-inflammatory effect. The search for new medicines and dietary supplements derived from plants have enhanced in the modern era. Ninety-one compounds of plant-derived drugs are in clinical trials as of 2007 [10, 11].

The following chapter will summarize the application of plant polyphenol against infectious diseases caused by bacteria and viruses as pathogens. It will describe in detail the diverse range of properties of various phenolics, with emphasis on the flavonoids, phenolic acids, Tannins and stilbenes with antimicrobial activity.

PLANT AS SOURCE OF ANTI-INFECTIVE AGENTS

Interest in the usage of plant medicine has been increased throughout the world in the past few years. Drugs derived from plant sources in the form of the traditional Ayurvedic and Chinese medicine have been used in the treatment of various human disorders for thousands of years. In developing countries, about 80% of the population use traditional medicinal plants as the initial source of medicine [12]. Furthermore, at least 25% of the modern pharmaceuticals contain compounds extracted from plant material or synthetic compounds based on isolated compounds from the plants [13]. Many natural product drugs (*e.g.* aspirin, quinine and morphine) are still in practice today [14, 15].

There are several reasons for using plants as a source of healing agents, such as to isolate biologically active compounds as a drug for direct use or to produce novel bio-active compounds that serve as lead compounds, and to use the plant extract in herbal medicine therapy [16]. The driving force for showing interest in the plant-derived antimicrobial agent is the ineffectiveness of traditional antibiotics; different resistance mechanisms evolved from bacteria, efflux pump susceptible antibiotics, toxic synthetic drugs against the newly emerging diseases, and the rapid rate of plant extinction [17].

Plants produce secondary metabolites (photosynthetic by-product or waste product), which are organic compounds and are not involved directly in the plant growth and development [18]. They are a large class of compounds that enable plants to interact with their environment and have physiological functions different from those of the primary metabolites [19]. Plant secondary metabolites play an important role in plant defence against herbivores [20], insects and microorganisms.

Medicinal plants are a rich source of secondary metabolites such as flavonoids, tannins, alkaloids, alkenyl phenols, lactones, terpenes, and terpenoids [21, 22]. Therefore, plants have been resisting the constant attacks of microorganisms by producing many secondary metabolites. On the other hand, micro-organisms are continuously trying to invade the plants by opposing the defensive actions of these compounds. According to this endless contest, the plant kingdom develops an enormous number of biochemical compounds for defense. The characterized plants based biochemical has been estimated to be at least 200,000 [23], which represents only a fraction of the compounds produced by the around 250,000 plant species growing on earth [23].

For many years, the plants were able to produce new and natural antimicrobials, and this made them succeed in fighting against microbes [24]. In the past, the early civilizations considered the plants as the main source of leads for antimicrobial and other medicines development [25]. This interest had led to the discovery of new bio active molecules by the pharmaceutical industry and the adoption of the public to the crude extracts of plants for self-medication. And, many plant extracts are reported to be used synergistically to enhance the activity of several traditional antibiotics [26, 27].

POLYPHENOLS

Polyphenols are natural compounds characterized by a high structural variety, and their existence in plants makes them an essential dietary component. They are not synthesized in humans or animals and can be found only in plants and certain fungal species [28]. Polyphenols are seen as secondary metabolites characterized by a high range of physiological functions [29, 30]. The human diet consists of a large part of plant-derived products, like vegetables, fruits and tea. These food products contain relatively high levels of polyphenols. Therefore, the average intake of polyphenols in a healthy human diet is expected to be at least 2-5 g/day [31]. Several studies have revealed that the high intake of polyphenols has protective effects against inflammatory diseases and cancer [32]. The anti-inflammatory effect of polyphenols is related to their antioxidant activity because of their scavenging and prevention of reactive oxygen and nitrogen species formation [33 - 36]. Phenolics are also reported to have antibacterial [37 - 41] anti-inflammatory [42], antidiabetic [43] and anti-viral properties [44]. Several medicinal plants are rich in polyphenols, which are classified as flavonoid drugs with much biological significance.

The main classes of polyphenol in nature are divided by their carbon skeleton; *i.e.*, the more common ones are phenolic acids and flavonoids, while the less common ones are stilbenes and lignans.

OCCURRENCE, STRUCTURES AND FUNCTIONS OF SIGNIFICANT POLYPHENOLS

Flavonoids

Most of the isolated polyphenols belong to the subclass flavonoids which are connected by a three-carbon bridge (C6–C3–C6) containing mostly 15 carbons.

Depending on the position of the linkage of the aromatic ring to the chromene moiety (Fig. **1**) this group can be divided into three classes; flavonoid, isoflavonoid and neoflavonoid (Fig. **1**).

They are categorised as compounds containing two or more aromatic rings, with one or more phenolic hydroxyl groups and are connected by a carbon bridge [45, 46].

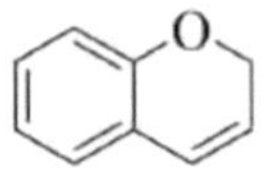

Chromene (Benzopyran)

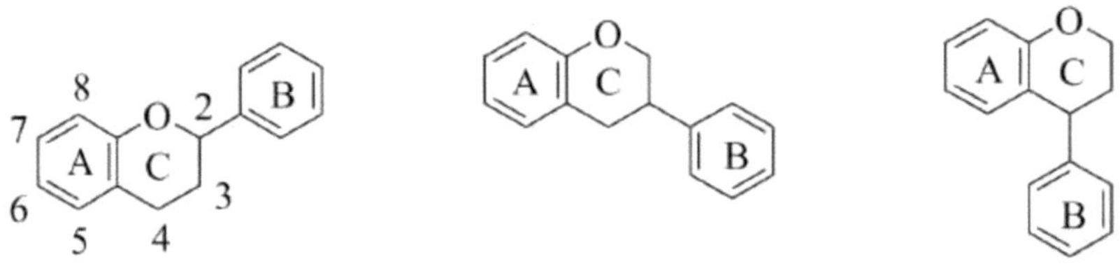

1 **2** **3**

Fig. (1). Representative structures of Flavonoid, iso-Flavonoid and neo-Flavonoid

Based on the degree of oxidation and saturation present in the C-ring, flavonoids are divided into subclasses, which are termed as flavonols (Fig. **2a**), flavanones (Fig. **2b**), flavones (Fig. **2c**), isoflavones (Fig. **2d**) , isoflavanes, flavanols (Fig. **2e**) and anthocyanidins. The flavanols are further subdivided into monomers and polymers (such as proanthocyanidins, theaflavins and thearubigins) [46].

Flavonoids, which are commonly present in nature as glycosides and partly as esters, rather than as aglycones, are the most abundant phenolics in our diets [47, 48]. Their occurrences are common to various foods, whereas sometimes restricted to a few foods stuff. For instance, soy contains genistein and daidzein as 1 mg/g of dry bean and known to be the main source for isoflavones [49]. On the other hand, the main source of flavanones is considered to be citrus fruits. For example, hesperidin is widely consumed (125–250 mg/L of juice) from oranges [50].

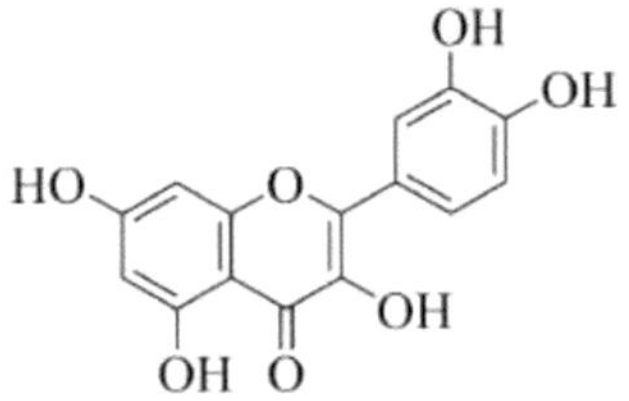

Quercetin

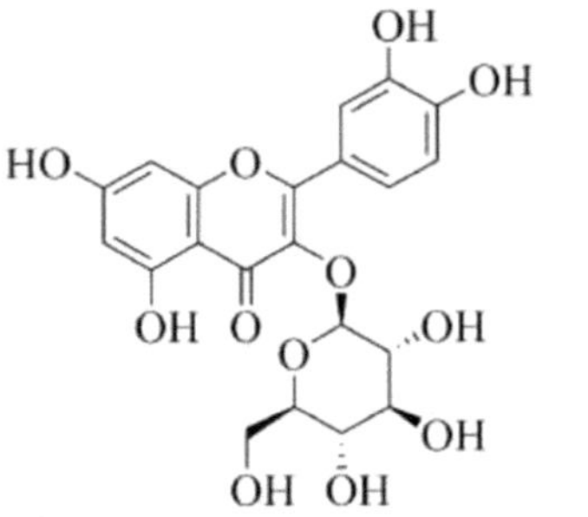

Quercetin 3-ß-D-glucoside

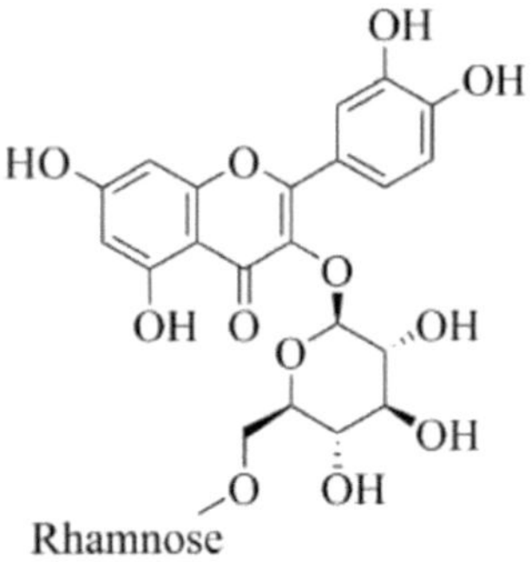

Rutin

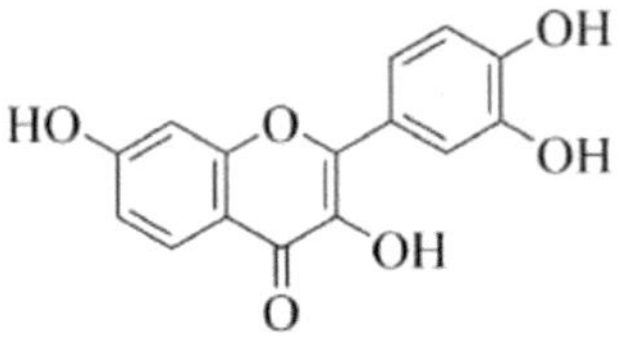

Fisetin

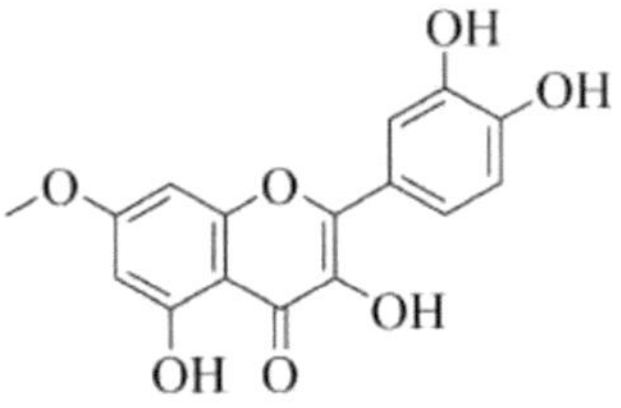

Rhamnetin

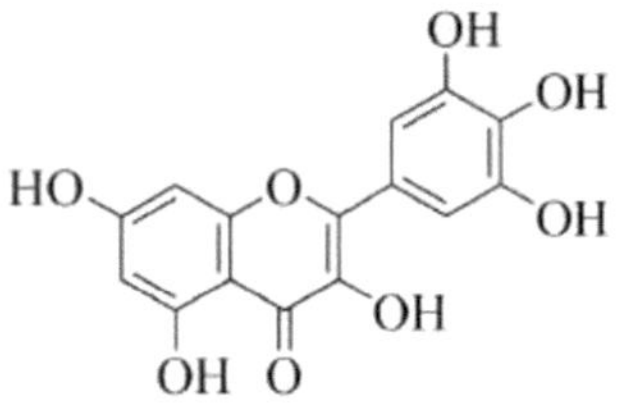

Myricetin

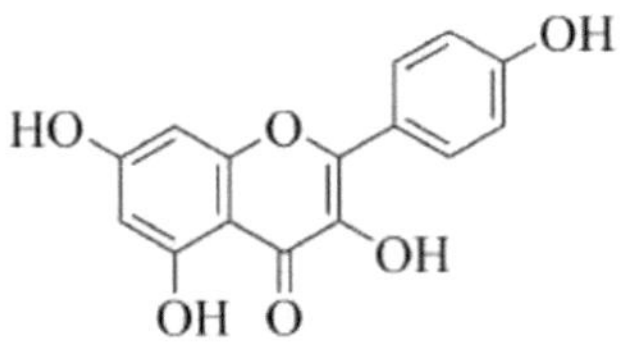

Kaempferol

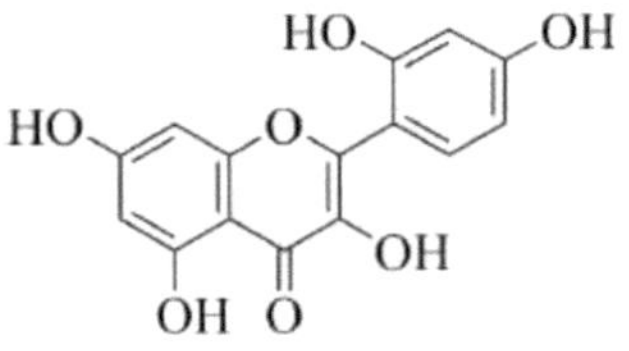

Morin

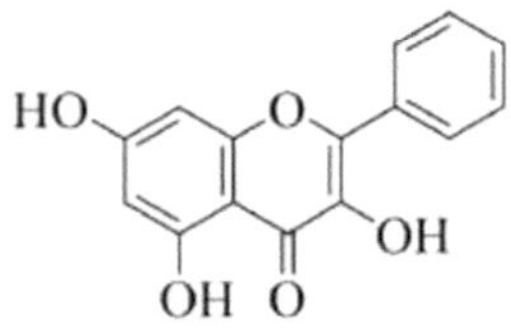

Galangin

Fig. (2a). Representative structures of Flavonols.

Quercetin is a commonly present flavonol in different diets as it is present in many fruits, vegetables and beverages. Onion is a rich source of quercetin (0.3mg/g of fresh leaves) followed by tea, which contains 10-25mg/L [51]. Flavones (luteolin and apigenin) are less common and present in celery and sweet red pepper [51]. The main flavan-3-ols are catechins. They are most abundant in green tea, which contains 1 g/L catechins [52]. Proanthocyanidins are polymeric flavanols, usually present in association with catechins and responsible for the astringency of food. The common sources are different fruits, beverages, as well as chocolate [53].

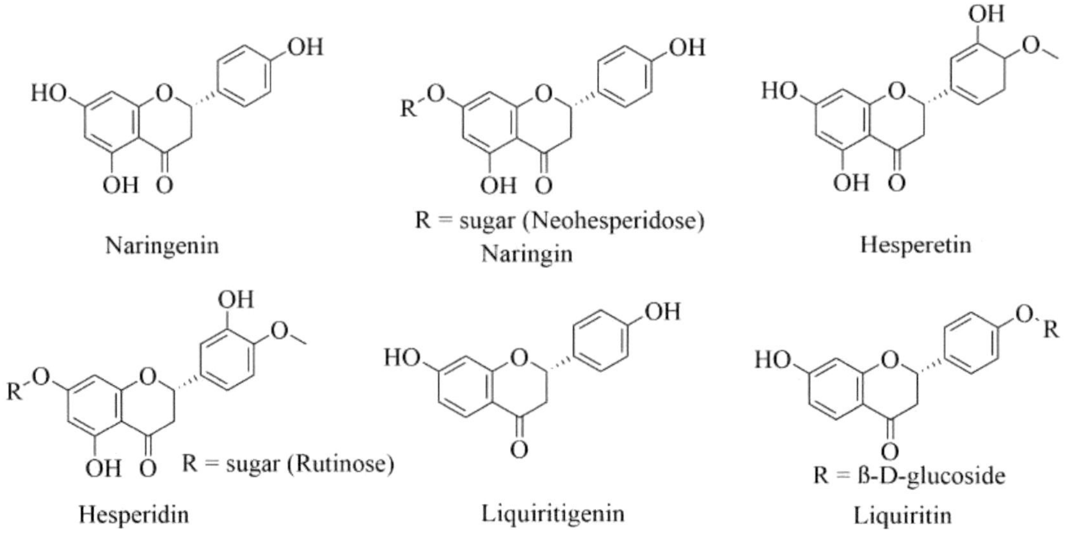

Fig. (2b). Representative structures of Flavanones.

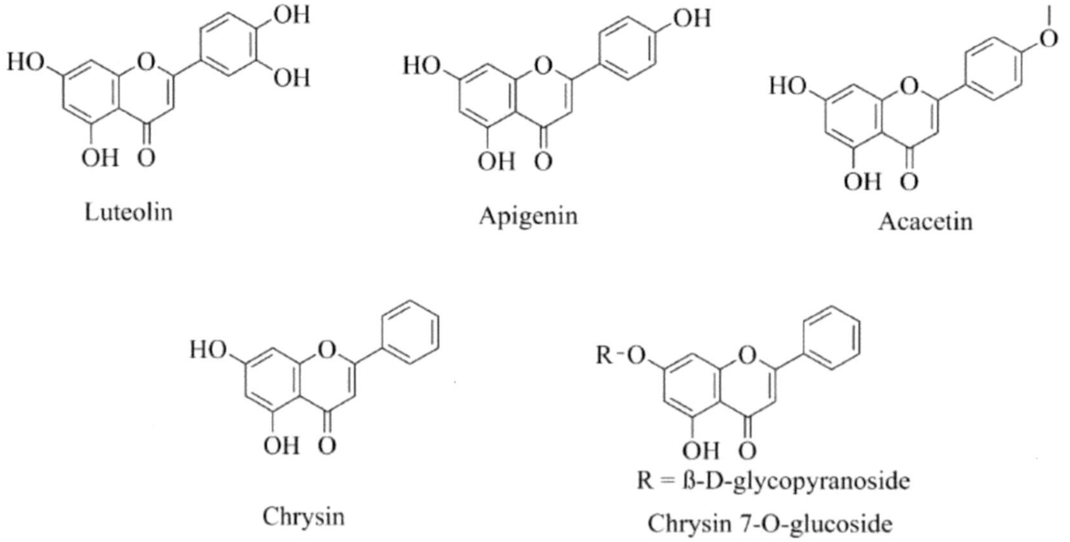

Fig. (2c). Representative structures of Flavones.

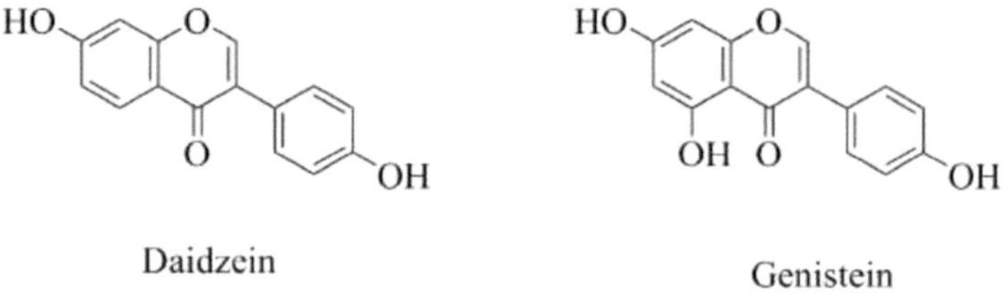

Fig. (2d). Representative structures of iso-Flavones.

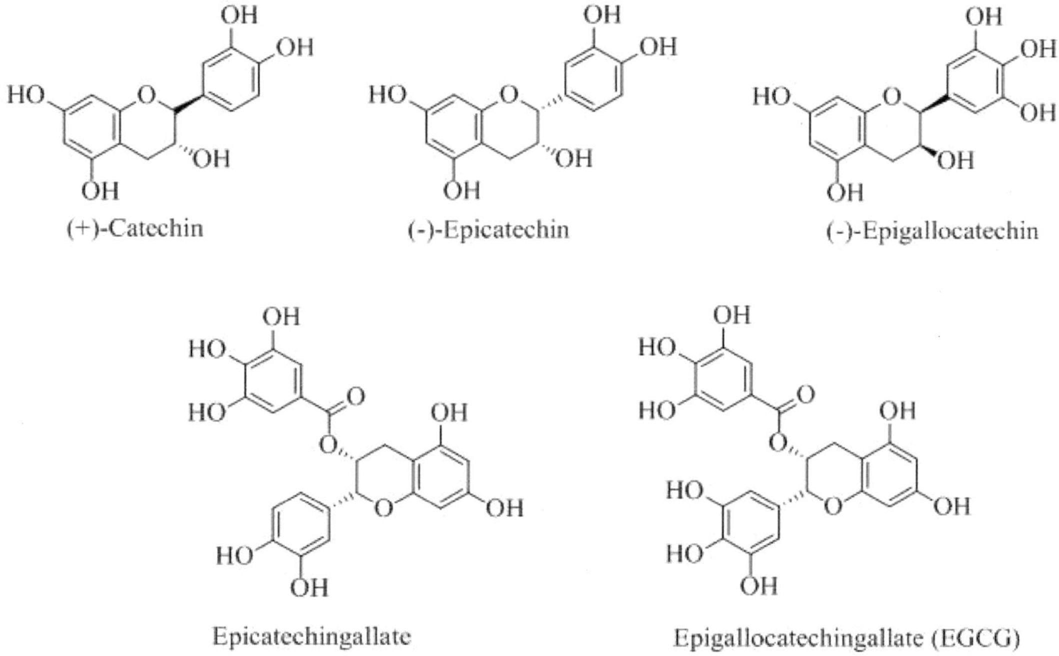

Fig. (2e). Representative structures of Flavanols (Flavan-3-ols).

Besides their role in plants as pigments or protection against UV, pathogens and herbivores, they are reported to have several biological effects such as antimicrobial activity [41], anti-inflammatory activities [54, 55] and antioxidant activity [56].

Phenolic Acids

Phenolic acids are further subdivided into derivatives of benzoic acid (C6-C1) and cinnamic acids (C6-C3) (Fig. **3**).

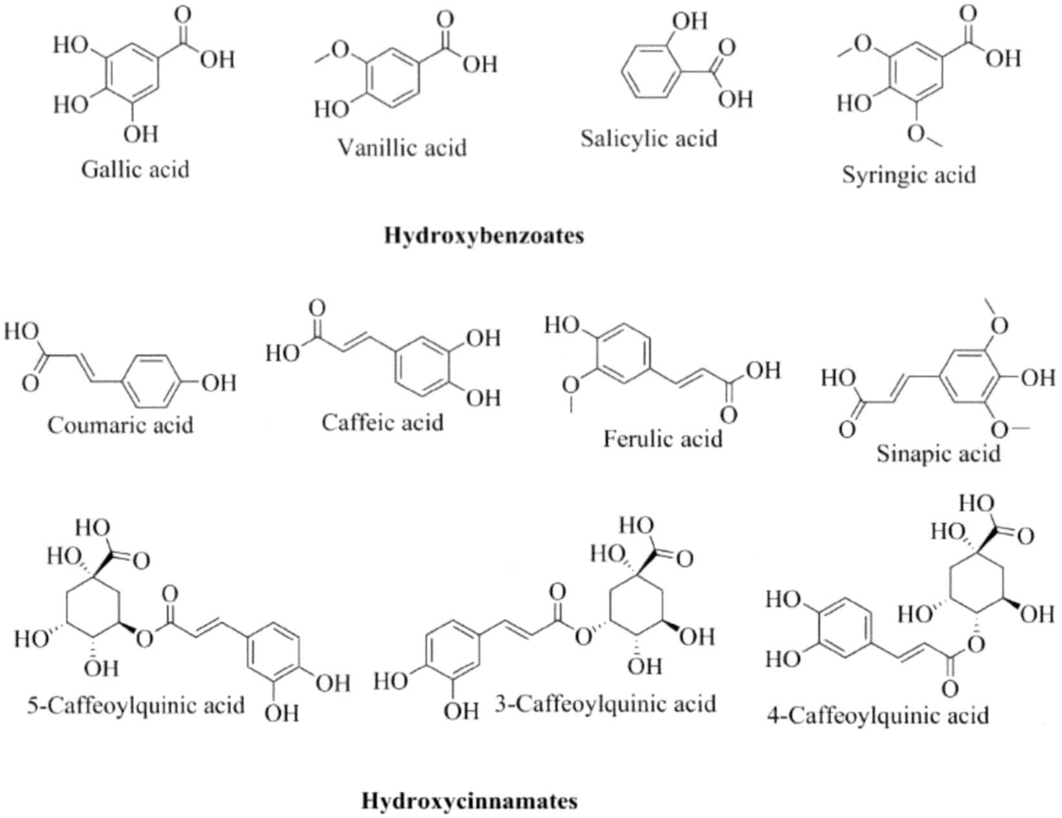

Fig. (3). Representative structures of Phenolic acids.

Hydroxybenzoic acid derivatives include acids such as gallic acid, ellagic acid, vanillic acid, salicylic acid and syringic acid. They are mostly found as free, esterified or glycosylated form. On the other hand, Hydroxycinnamic acids are mainly present as ester, amides or found in the glycosylated form. It includes acids such as caffeic, *p*-coumaric, ferulic and sinapic acids. The best example of phenolic acid is caffeic acid and ferulic acid. Both can be formed in the form of esters. Wheat bran is a rich source of ferulic acid (5mg/kg) [57]. The hydroxycinnamic acids (*i.e*., caffeic, p-coumaric, and ferulic acid.) form esters with quinic acid, which are commonly referred to as chlorogenic acids. Coffee is a rich source of chlorogenic acids, where one cup of instant coffee (200 ml) contains 50–150 mg of chlorogenic acid [58]. Many fruits and vegetables consist of caffeic acid and coffee consist of chlorogenic acid [58]. Chlorogenic acids have a broad range of biological activities, such as anti-bacterial [59], antiviral [60], anti-fungal [61] and anti-inflammatory [62].

Tannins

Tannins are a group of polyphenols, which are subdivided into condensed and hydrolysable tannins (Fig. **4**) , varies from 500 to 3,000 *m/z* range.

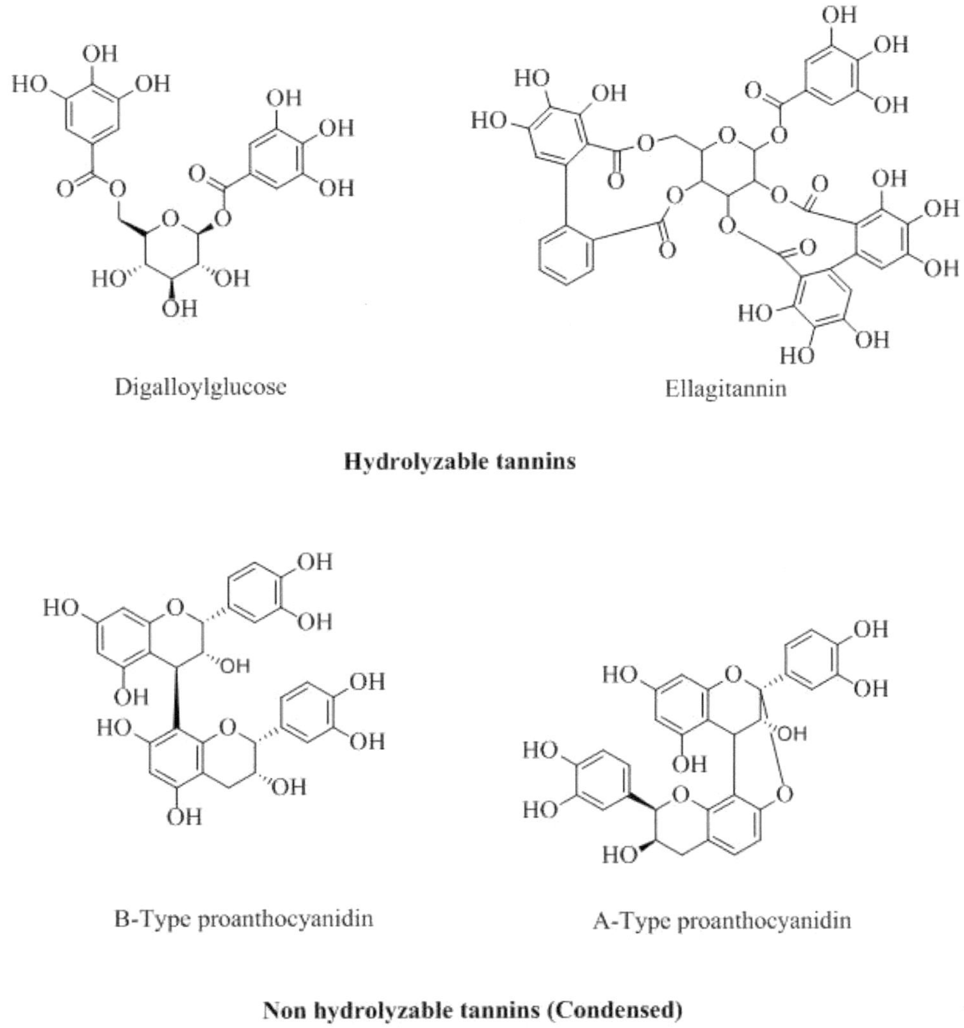

Fig. (4). Representative structures of Tannins.

They are mostly present as polymers and commonly form complexes with polysaccharides alkaloids and particularly with proteins [63]. The hydrolysable tannins are esters of sugars, gallic acid and ellagic acid such as digalloylglucose and ellagitannin, which are the best examples of hydrolysable tannin. While the non-hydrolysable or condensed tannins are usually flavan-3-ol oligomers and polymers known as proanthocyanidins [64]. Proanthocyanidins are known as condensed tannins, having a wide range of structures and molecular weights, and this makes their amounts estimation difficult in plants [63, 65]. Tannins are astringent and bitter substances and responsible for the astringent taste of fruits [66]. The level of astringency changes over maturation and often disappears when the fruit reaches ripeness. They are mostly found in fruits and vegetables such as pomegranate, strawberry, raspberry, grape, blackberry, peach, olive, plum, chick pea and lentil. Other sources of tannins are cocoa, chocolate, tea, red wine, cider and coffee. Tannins have various biological effects since they are antioxidants, potential metal ion chelators, protein precipitating agents [67], as well as reported to have antibacterial [68] and antiviral activities [69].

Stilbenes and Lignans

Stilbenes (C6-C2-C6), such as resveratrol (Fig. **5**), piceid and viniferin are phytoalexins produced by plants in response to disease, injury, and stress [70]. They are found in small quantities in Vitaceae plant family, which includes grapes. Low amount of these phenolics are present in the human diet such as is resveratrol. Several studies have reported that resveratrol is known to have anti-carcinogenic and coronary-protective properties. However, the low dietary concentration is not sufficient for the significant effects [71, 72]. Moreover, the anti-inflammatory, antioxidant [73] and antibacterial [74] activities of stilbenes were also reported.

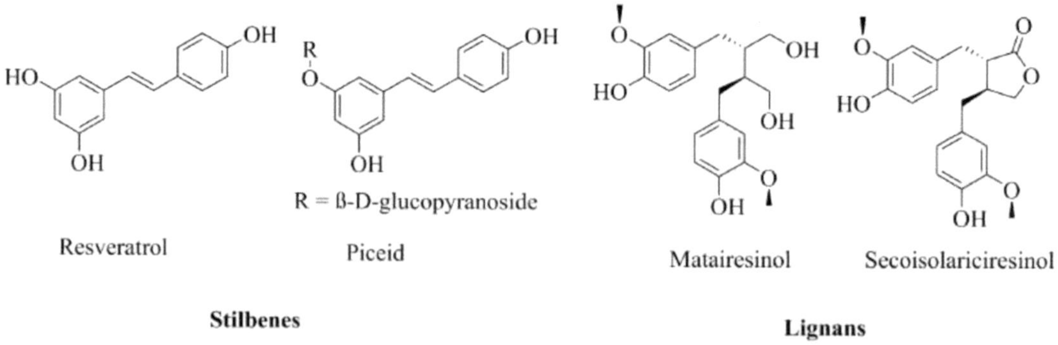

Fig. (5). Representative structures of Stilbenes and Lignans.

Lignans (Fig. **5**) are plant secondary metabolites consist of two phenylpropanoid units [75] and considered as abundant class of phenolic compounds found in woods. Lignans are also found in small quantities in some fruits (pears), vegetables (carrots and garlic), leguminous plants (lentils) and cereals [65]. Representative examples of this class of compounds are secoisolariciresinol and matairesinol. They are known to have protective effects in plants and have anti-cancer and chemo-protective properties. They are reported to be used in treatments for cancer, lymphoma and leukemia [75, 76].

BIOSYNTHESIS OF POLYPHENOLS

The biosynthetic pathways of polyphenols reported in the literature are pentose phosphate, mevalonic acid, shikimate, and phenylpropanoids, where various polyphenols are biosynthesized [77 - 79]. Flavonoids, stilbenes, and phenolic acids biosynthesis mainly occur through shikimic acid pathway. The shikimate pathway is known to produce phenylalanine and cinnamic acid as metabolites. The transformation of phenylalanine to cinnamate is catalyzed by PAL (phenylalanine ammonia lyase) enzyme. The cinnamate further produces p-coumaroyl-CoA, which reacts with malonyl-CoA molecules. Further biosynthesis of flavonoids is initiated by chalcone synthase (CHS) enzyme, resulting in chalcone. Chalcones are not the end-product of the pathway, but it proceeds with several further enzymatic steps to produce other classes of flavonoids (*i.e.*, flavanones, dihydroflavonols, anthocyanins, isoflavones, flavones, pro-anthocyanidins (PA) and flavonols, which represent the side branches of the mentioned flavonoids biosynthetic pathway [78].

BIOAVAILABILITY, UPTAKE AND METABOLISM OF POLYPHENOLS BY GUT MICROBIOTA

The bioavailability and bioactivity of dietary and plant phenolics usually depend upon the difference between original chemical structures and newly produced modified metabolite. The major portion of the plant and dietary phenolics are modified during absorption; however, very small amount of the absorbed phenolics retain their original structure [80, 81]. Most modification occurs by intestinal microbiota through conversion and transformation in the colon before absorption. The intestinal and colonic conversion of phenolics is sometimes essential for their absorption, which modulates their biological activity as well [82]. Therefore, the gut, especially colon is considered as an active site for metabolism which requires further attention.

Gut bacteria can carry out several processes that hydrolyze glycosides, glucuronides, amides, sulfates, esters, and lactones. Ring-cleavage, reduction, decarboxylation, demethylation, and dehydroxylation reactions are also carried out by Gut bacteria [51]. The hydrolysis of glycosides ends in metabolites, which are potentially more active than their parent compounds. The aglycons are further converted by bacteria to produce more or less bio-active compounds. It depends on the products being formed and the substrate being metabolized [83]. On the other hand, phenolic compounds can interact with the gut microbiota, as they are also antimicrobial, which modulates the microbial inhabitants of the gastrointestinal (GI) tract. They both have effects on gastrointestinal health and also in the metabolism of dietary phenolics [84].

Data on bioavailability and uptake of polyphenol metabolites are still very scarce [80, 85]. Additionally, complete intestinal mechanism of GIT absorption of polyphenol substances is still unknown.

ANTIBACTERIAL ACTIVITY OF POLYPHENOLS

Many research groups have reported antimicrobial activity of purified natural product and crude extracts of plants rich in polyphenols. Antibacterial activities of flavonoids are divided based on differences in their backbone structure into subclasses such as flavonols, flavanols, flavanones, flavones and isoflavones. The minimum inhibitory concentrations (MICs) of phenolics against different bacteria are presented in Table **1**.

Antibacterial Activity of Flavonols

Flavonols possess a remarkable activity against several Gram-positive (*Actinomyces naeslundii* and *Staphylococcus aureus*) and Gram-negative bacteria *(Prevotella species, Escherichia coli*, *Porphyromonas gingivalis*, and Fusobacterium nucleatum), due to their different mechanisms of action [86, 87]. Among flavonols, the most responsible compound for antibacterial activity is quercetin, kaempferol and myricetin [88 - 93]. The most likely antibacterial effect of quercetin and other flavonols is inhibition of DNA gyrase enzyme (*i.e.*; in *Escherichia coli*) [94]. In *in-vitro* assays, quercetin is reported to display an important antibacterial feature by dissipating bacterial membrane potential and diminished the cell motility [95]. Liu *et al.* [91] showed that quercetin aglycones exhibited strong antibacterial activity against *Staphylococcus aureus* and *Staphylococcus haemolyticus.*

Lee *et al.* [90] reported the effects of quercetin against *Escherichia coli*, while Siriwong *et al.* [96] have assessed the antibacterial effect of both quercetin and luteolin against *Streptococcus pyogenes*. In another study, rhamnetin, myricetin, morin, and quercetin showed strong antibacterial activity against Gram-negative pathogen (*Chlamydia pneumonia*); the infectivity was decreased by 50% compared to controls using the polyphenol concentrations ranging from 0.5 to 50 mM [97]. Moreover, rhamnetin was observed to be more active than quercetin and morin, possibly due to the methoxy group in the A-ring, which gives a hydrophobic nature to this molecule [97]. Many other research groups have reported that flavonols possess antibacterial activity. Few examples of such falvonols are quercetin, 3-*O*-methyl quercetin and various quercetin glycosides, kaempferol and its derivatives [98 - 105], other flavonols [104, 106, 107] and flavonol glycosides [108 - 111].

Antibacterial Activity of Flavan-3-Ols

Flavan-3-ols is a group of flavonoids consisting of catechin, epicatechin, gallocatechin, epigallocatechin, and the corresponding gallate esters. EGCG (epigallocatechin gallate) exerting most antibacterial actions by several modes against *Staphylococcus* (*i.e*., damage to the cell membrane [112], a decrease in slime production [113], as well as have the ability of neutralization of enterotoxin B [114]. The antibacterial activity of tea *(Camellia sinensis)* catechins and their gallates is known since the 1990s, which inhibited the growth of several bacterial species, such as *Vibrio cholerae, Streptococcus mutans, Clostridium perfringes,* and *Escherichia coli* in *in-vitro* studies [115 - 118].

Several other studies have shown the tea polyphenols against *Staphylococcus aureus* [119, 120], *Serratia marcescens* [121], *Pseudomonas aeruginosa* [122, 123] and *Helicobacter pylori* [124, 125]. Among all catechins, EGCG is the most abundant catechin exhibiting strong bactericidal action against *Staphylococcus aureus*, *Streptococcus pyogenes*, coagulase negative *staphylococci* and *Streptococcus mutans* [126 - 128].

Lee and Tan [129] have reported the MIC and MBC values of EGCG against *Enterococcus faecalis,* which were 5μg/mL and 20μg/mL, respectively. Other groups also reported the killing action of EGCG against *Streptococcus pyogenes* [130], *Bacillus, Clostridium* [131], *Salmonella typhi* [128] and *Escherichia coli* [132]. The MIC required to inhibit the growth of 90% of clinical isolates of *Helicobacter pylori* organisms was found to be 100 mg/mL [133]. On the other hand, some researcher described mild activity of EGCG against Gram-negative strains such as *Escherichia coli* [112, 134, 135] *Salmonella typhi* [128] and *Pseudomonas aeruginosa.*

EGCG also inhibited the growth of imipenem-resistant *Klebsiella pneumoniae* at 300–650μg/mL, as demonstrated by Cho *et al.* [136]. In particular, EGCG at sub-MIC concentration did not affect *Escherichia coli* (O157: H7) growth rate but showed a significant anti-pathogenic effect [132]. Researchers have also reported the synergism between other agents and flavonoids against resistant strains of bacteria [137 - 139].

Table 1. Minimum inhibitory concentration of Polyphenols classes against Gram-positive and Gram-negative bacteria observed by different groups.

Flavonol				
Compound	**Antibacterial Spectrum**	**MIC/ MBC (µg/mL)**	**MIC (µM)**	**Reference**
Quercetin	*Staphylococcus aureus*	6.25		[91]
	Escherichia coli	31.25		[273]
	Escherichia coli KL-16, *Salmonella typhimurium, Pseudomonas maltophilia, Staphylococcus epidermidis* and *Staphylococcus aureus*	>125		[273]
	Staphylococcus haemolyticus	50		[91]
	Streptococcus pyogenes	128		[96]
	Bacillus cereus	350		[100]
	Salmonella enteritidis	250		
	Mycobacterium phlei	>I00		[105]
	Pseudomonas aeruginosa PA01	>128		[89]
	Escherichia coli K-12	64		
	Escherichia coli DNA gyrase		0.14 ± 0.04	
	Escherichia coli topoIV		6.42± 0.07	
	methicillin-resistant *Staphylococcus aureus*	>128		
	Escherichia coli TG1	>1000		[274]
	Escherichia coli W3310	>1000		[275]
	Escherichia coli, Klebsiella pneumonia, Enterobacter aerogenes and *Enterobacter cloacae*	512 (MBC)		[99]
	Staphylococcus aureus, Proteus vulgaris and *Pseudomonas aeruginosa,*	256 (MBC)		

(Table 1) cont.....

Quercetin-3-O-Glucoside	*Escherichia coli* W3310	>2000		[275]
	Bacillus cereus	350		[100]
	Salmonella enteritidis	300		
Rutin	*Mycobacterium phlei*	>I00		[105]
	Escherichia coli, Proteus vulgaris and *Pseudomonas aeruginosa*,	64		[99]
	Klebsiella pneumonia, Enterobacter aerogenes and *Enterobacter cloacae*	128		
	Staphylococcus aureus	16		
Fisetin	*Staphylococcus epidermidis*	100		[104]
	Mycobacterium phlei	>I00		[105]
Rhamnetin	*Chlamydophila pneumoniae*		50	[97]
Isorhamnetin 3-O-Robinobioside	*Mycobacterium phlei*	50		[105]
Myricetin	*Chlamydophila pneumoniae*		29	[97]
	Staphylococcus epidermidis	100		[104]
	Escherichia coli	62.5		[273]
	Escherichia coli KL-16, *Salmonella typhimurium, Pseudomonas maltophilia* and *Staphylococcus aureus*	>125		
	Staphylococcus epidermidis	>62.5		
Kaempferol	*Staphylococcus epidermidis*	50		[104]
	Mycobacterium phlei	50		[105]
4',5,7-Tri-0-Methylkaempferol	*Mycobacterium phlei*	>I00		
Morin	*Chlamydophila pneumoniae*		50	[97]
	Bacillus cereus	300		[100]
	Salmonella enteritidis	150		
	Mycobacterium phlei	>I00		
Morin-3-O-Lyxoside	*Bacillus cereus*	250		
	Salmonella enteritidis	200		
	Bacillus cereus	300		
	Salmonella enteritidis	200		
Galangin	*Staphylococcus epidermidis*	6.3		[104]

(Table 1) cont.....

Flavanone				
Compound	**Antibacterial Spectrum**	**MIC/ MBC** (μg/mL)	**MIC** (μM)	**Reference**
Naringenin	*Escherichia coli* K12, *Pseudomonas aeruginosa* PAOI, and methicillin-resistant *Staphylococcus aureus*	>I28		[170]
	Escherichia coli TG1	>1000		[274]
	Helicobacter pylori	80		[153]
Naringen	*Helicobacter pylori*	>I00		
Hesperidin	*Escherichia coli* and *Klebsiella pneumonia*	128		[99]
	Pseudomonas aeruginosa, *Enterobacter aerogenes* and *Enterobacter cloacae*	64		
	Aeromonas hydrophila	3125		[152]
	Helicobacter pylori	>I00		[153]
	Helicobacter pylori	80		
Liquiritin	*Escherichia coli* K12, *Pseudomonas aeruginosa* PAOI, and methicillin-resistant *Staphylococcus aureus*	>I28		[170]
Liquiritigenin	*Escherichia coli* K12, *Pseudomonas aeruginosa* PAOI, and methicillin-resistant *Staphylococcus aureus*	>I28		

Flavone				
Compound	**Antibacterial Spectrum**	**MIC/ MBC** (μg/mL)	**MIC** (μM)	**Reference**
Luteolin	*Streptococcus pyogenes*	128		[96]
	Chlamydophila pneumoniae		8.8	[97]
	Staphylococcus aureus, *Staphylococcus haemolyticus*	50		[91]
	Escherichia coli, *Xanthomonas vesicatoria*, *Magnaporthe oryzae*	I00		
	Agrobacterium tumefacien, *Pseudomonas lachryman*, *Bacillus subtilis*,	200		

(Table 1) cont.....

Apigenin	*Escherichia coli, Klebsiella pneumonia, Proteus vulgaris, Pseudomonas aeruginosa,*	64		[99]
	Enterobacter aerogenes Enterobacter cloacae	128		
	Staphylococcus aureus	32		
	Mycoeacterium phlei	>I00		[105]
Acacetin	*Chlamydophila pneumoniae*		29	[97]
Chrysin	*Staphylococcus aureus, E. coli*	6.25		[91]
	Agrobacterium tumefaciens, Bacillus subtilis and *Staphylococcus haemolyticus*	12.5		
	Magnaporthe oryzae	50		
Chrysin 7-O-d-Glucopyranoside	*Staphylococcus aureus, Escherichia coli,* Agrobacterium tumefaciens, *Bacillus subtilis* and *Staphylococcus haemolyticus*	150–400		
Isoflavanones				
Compound	**Antibacterial Spectrum**	**MIC/ MBC** (μg/mL)	**MIC** (μM)	**Reference**
Daidzein	Vancomycin-resistant *Enterococcus faecalis*	16		[169]
	Salmonella typhimurium, Bacillus subtilis, Escherichia coli, Pseudomonas aeruginosa, Proteus vulgaris and *Staphylococcus aureus*	64		
	Oxacillin-resistant *Staphylococcus aureus*	128		
	methicillin-resistantStaphylococcus aureus	128		[170, 172]
Genistein	Vancomycin-resistant *Enterococcus faecalis*	32		[169]
	Salmonella typhimurium, Bacillus subtilis, Escherichia coli, Pseudomonas aeruginosa, Proteus vulgaris and *Staphylococcus aureus*	64		
	Oxacillin-resistant *Staphylococcus aureus*	128		
Flavanol				
Compound	**Antibacterial Spectrum**	**MIC/ MBC** (μg/mL)	**MIC** (μM)	**Reference**

(Table 1) cont.....

Epigallocatechin gallate	Methicillin-resistant *Staphylococcus aureus* strains		140-280	[126]
	Staphylococcus aureus		560	
	Vancomycin-Intermediate *Staphylococcus aureus* Mu50		280	
	Escherichia coli K12	> 400		[276]
	Escherichia coli O157:H7	100-500		[112]
	Escherichia coli	400		[135]
	Pseudomonas aeruginosa	200-400		
	Pseudomonas aeruginosa	500		[112]
	Streptococcus mutans	100		
	Staphylococcus aureus	50-100		
	Enterococcus faecalis	5		[129]
	Porphyromonas gingivalis	500-5000		[277]
	Klebsiella pneumoniae	300-650		[136]
	Helicobacter pylori various *strains*	1–64		[124]
	Geobacillus stearothermophilus and *Bacillus coagulans*	100		[131]
	Clostridium thermoaceticum	>400		
Epigallocatechin	*Staphylococcus epidermidis*	50		[104]
	Helicobacterpylori various strains	8–256		[124]
Epicatechin Gallate	*Helicobacter pylori* various strains	1–256		
Catechin	*Escherichia coli* TG1	>1000		[274]
Phenolic Acids				
Compound	**Antibacterial Spectrum**	**MIC/ MBC** (μg/mL)	**MIC** (μM)	**Reference**
Chlorogenic Acid	*Streptococcus pneumoniae*	20		[59]
	Staphylococcus aureus, *Bacillus subtilis*, and *Salmonella typhimurium*	40		
	Escherichia coli and *Shigella dysenteriae*	80		
	Escherichia coli O157:H7 and *Listeria innocua*		1000-25000	[176]
	Escherichia coli, *Pseudomonas aeruginosa*, *Staphylococcus aureus*, *Enterococcus faecium*, and *Proteus vulgaris*	10		[177]
	Klebsiella pneumoniae	5		
Tannins				
Compound	**Antibacterial Spectrum**	**MIC/ MBC** (μg/mL)	**MIC** (μM)	**Reference**

(Table 1) cont.....

Proanthocyanidins	*Escherichia coli* O157:H7		500	[190]
	Listeria monocytogenes,		250	
Condensed Tannins	*Escherichia coli* ATCC 35352 and ATCC 25922	20-40		[191]
	E. coli O157:H7 3081, H4420N, E318N, EDL933, R508N2006	20-50		
Ellagic Acid	*Moraxella catarrhalis*	15		[192]
	Corynebacterium diphtheriae	30		
	Neisseria meningitides, *Bacillus subtilis*, *Clostridium sporogenes*	60		
	Helicobacter pylori	125		
	Staphylococcus aureus	500		
	Streptococcus group A, B and G, *Streptococcus pneumonia, Enterococcus faecalis, Staphylococcus epidermidis*, Haemophilus influenza, Klebsiella pneumoniae	> 1000		
Gallotannin (1, 2, 6-tri-O-Galloyl-β-d-Glucopyranose)	*Escherichia coli*, *Staphylococcus aureus*, *Escherichia coli*, (ATCC 8739)	12.1-97.5		[194]
	Klebsiella pneumonia; S. aureus (ATCC 6538P)	24.3-97.5		
	Pseudomonas aeruginosa	48·7–195		
Ellagintannins (Sanguiin H6)	*Corynebacterium diphtheriae*	30		[192]
	Staphylococcus epidermidis	125		
	Staphylococcus aureus	250		
	Streptococcus group A,Streptococcus pneumonia, Bacillus subtilis; Moraxella catarrhalis	500		
	Streptococcus group B and G, *Enterococcus faecalis, Neisseria meningitides, Haemophilus influenza, Helicobacter pylori*, Klebsiella pneumoniae	> 1000		
Stilbenes				
Compound	**Antibacterial Spectrum**	**MIC/ MBC** (μg/mL)	**MIC** (μM)	**Reference**

(Table 1) cont.....

Gnemonol	Methicillin-resistant *Staphylococcus aureus* strains	6.25		[202]
	Vancomycin-resistant *Enterococci*	12.5		
Gnetin E	Methicillin-resistant *Staphylococcus aureus* strains	25		
	Vancomycin-resistant *Enterococci*	12.5		
Hemsleyanol D	Methicillin-resistant *Staphylococcus aureus*	2		[203]
Genetin E	Methicillin-resistant *Staphylococcus aureus*	4		
Combretastatin B5 (2',3',4-trihydroxyl-3,5,-'-trimethoxybibenzyl)	*Staphylococcus aureus*	16		[204]
	Pseudomonas aeruginosa, Enterococcus faecalis	125		
	Escherichia coli	> 250		

Antibacterial Activity of Flavanones

The antimicrobial activity of flavanones [140 - 144], naringenin, hesperidin and hesperetin [145 - 148] of flavanones subclass have been reported by many groups. Naringenin was found to be active against *Salmonella typhimurium* [149] and *Pseudomonas aeruginosa* [150]. Hesperidin has been described and found to be active against *Staphylococcus aureus* [151] and *Aeromonas hydrophylia* [152]. In addition to the inhibitory activity against *Staphylococcus aureus*, hesperetin and hesperidin were also reported to be active against *Helicobacter pylori* [151, 153].

Antibacterial Activity Flavones

These flavonoids (luteolin, apigenin and chrysin) share the 2-phenylchromen-4-one backbone. Many studies have reported the antibacterial action of luteolin and luteolin-7- glucoside [154 - 156], other flavones [157 - 160], flavone glycosides [108], apigenin, luteolin and chrysin [161 - 165] against both Gram-positive and Gram-negative bacteria. Liu *et al.* [91] have shown that chrysin was active against *Staphylococcus aureus*, *Escherichia coli* at MIC of 6.25μg/mL and also inhibited the growth of *Agrobacterium tumefaciens, Bacillus subtilis and Staphylococcus haemolyticus* at one fold higher concentration. Luteolin showed less antibacterial activity than chrysin against the mentioned bacterial strains (MIC range 50-200 μg/mL) in the same study. Moreover, luteolin is reported to be active against *Staphylococcus aureus*, Bacillus subtilis, Pseudomonas fluorescens and *Escherichia coli* [91, 166, 167].

Antibacterial Activity of Isoflavones

One of the most active isoflavones is daidzein, where studies concerning the antimicrobial activity of isoflavones have been described [142, 168]. Genistein and daidzein were found to be effective against different bacteria, the most active compound *in vitro* was daidzein (MIC range was 16–128μg/mL), where the most susceptible strain was vancomycin-resistant *Enterococcus faecalis* among other bacteria [169].

Other groups have reported inhibition of *Staphylococcus aureus* (MRSA strains) by Genistein and various other Isoflavones at a concentration range of 16-128g/mL [170 - 172]. The antibacterial actions are assumed to be due to inhibition of topoisomerase IV enzyme of bacteria [173].

Antibacterial Activity of Phenolic Acids

Pure phenolic acids, such as hydroxycinnamic acids are reported to have bacteriostatic and bactericidal effect against numerous strains of *Listeria monocytogenes* [174]. Caffeic, *p*-coumaric and ferulic acids also showed activity against Gram-negative (*Escherichia coli*) and gram-positive bacteria (*i.e.*, *Staphylococcus aureus*) [175]. Chlorogenic acids, an esterified form of hydroxycinnamic acids, have a broad range of biological activities, such as anti-bacterial [59], antiviral [60] and anti-fungal [61].

Chlorogenic acid inhibited the growth (by >90%) of *Escherichia coli* (O157:H7) and *Listeria innocua* with the comparison to the control [176]. Moreover, Chlorogenic acid is also reported to be active against *Escherichia coli*, Shigella dysenteriae, Streptococcus pneumoniae and *Salmonella typhimurium*, respectively [59].

Bajko *et al.* [177] have recently shown the antibacterial effect of 5-O-caffeoylquinic acid against *Escherichia coli*, *Pseudomonas aeruginosa*, *Staphylococcus aureus*, Klebsiella pneumonia, Enterococcus faecium and *Proteus vulgaris*. Out of tested organism, 5-CQA was found to possess the strongest antimicrobial activity against *Klebsiella pneumonia*.

On the other hand, according to Puupponen-PimiaÈ *et al.* [178], phenolic acids (cinnamic acids and chlorogenic acid) showed activity against gram-negative bacteria only at high concentrations (500 μg well^{-1}), where chlorogenic acid was the weakest inhibitor against *Escherichia coli* (CM 871).

Dogazaki *et al.* [179] and Furuhata *et al.* [180] have reported the antibacterial activity of brewed coffee against a strain of *Legionella pneumophila*, where the identified active substances were caffeic, chlorogenic, and protocatechuic acids. The reported MIC values of chlorogenic acid against various gram-positive and gram-negative bacteria are presented in Table **1** of this article.

Antibacterial Activity of Tannins

Many traditional medicinal plants which are rich in Tannins were reported to have antimicrobial compounds [181, 182]. Both condensed (proanthocyanidins) and hydrolyzable (gallotannins and ellagitannins) tannins are described with numerous antimicrobial activities (MIC values are in Table **1**. Proanthocyanidin was shown to prevent adhesion and reduced biofilm production by a variety of pathogens including *Pseudomonas aerugionosa*, *Escherichia coli* and other microorganisms [183 - 186].

The Proanthocyanidins isolated from berries inhibited the growth of several pathogenic bacteria, such as *Streptococcus mutans, Escherichia coli*, *Helicobacter pylori*, *Listeria monocytogenes*, Salmonella typhimurium, and oxacillin-resistant *Staphylococcus aureus* [68, 187 - 190].

Liu *et al.* [191] have studied *Dalea purpurea*'s condensed tannins, where they have shown the inhibitory activity of proanthocyanidins against *Escherichia coli* at low inhibitory concentrations (20-50 μg/ml).

Hydrolysable tannins are also well known for their antimicrobial activity, where ellagitannins displayed the inhibitory activity against *Salmonella, Staphylococcus, Helicobacter, Escherichia coli*, Clostridium, Campylobacter and *Bacillus* species [178]. Krauze-Baranowska *et al.* [192] have tested Sanguiin H-6 (Ellagitannins), which exhibited bactericidal activity against *Streptococcus group A, Streptococcus pneumoniae, Corynebacterium diphtheria* and *Staphylococcus epidermidis*. It also inhibited *Bacillus subtilis, Clostridium sporogenes, Staphylococcus aureus* and *Moraxella catarrhali* species. In the same study, it was shown that ellagic acid also showed the same activity against many strains as sanguiin H-6. However, there was no antimicrobial activity displayed against *Streptococcus pneumoniae* and *Staphylococcus epidermidis* but displayed inhibitory activity against *Neisseria meningitides.* Furthermore, their research confirmed the ellagic acid activity towards *Helicobacter pylori*, while dimeric sanguiin H-6 did not exhibit any antimicrobial activity against *Helicobacter pylori*. The Minimum inhibitory concentration of sanguiin H-6 and ellagic acid against mentioned bacterial strains are indicated in Table **1** .

Gallotannins are also reported to possess antimicrobial activity against various gram-positive (such as *Staphylococcus*, *Bacillus subtilis, Bacillus cereus, Clostridium botulinum* and *Campylobacter jejuni*) and gram-negative bacteria (such as *Escherichia coli* and *Salmonella enterica* [193]. Bag *et al.* [194], has reported as gallotannin (1, 2, 6-tri-O-galloyl-β-d-glucopyranose) isolated from *Terminalia chebula* fruit which possesses intense antibacterial activity against multi drugs resistant bacteria (*i.e.*, *Pseudomonas aeruginosa*, *Escherichia coli*, Klebsiella pneumoniae and *Staphylococcus aureus*).

Antibacterial Activity of Stilbenes

Stilbenes, especially resveratrol is known to have anti-carcinogenic effect with unique forms of cell death induction in a variety of tumor cells [195]. Beside the chemo-preventive properties of stilbenes, many authors have reported the antibacterial activities of stilbenes [196 - 199].

Resveratrol inhibited *cholera* toxin [74] and inhibited virulence factor expression in wild-type strains of *Proteus mirabilis* [200]. Augustine *et al.* [201] have also reported that antimicrobial activity of resveratrol against *Vibrio cholerae* and inhibited biofilm formation.

Sakagami *et al.* [202] have reported two resveratrol trimmers (gnemonol B and gnetin E) obtained from the Gnetum species, which were found to exhibit strong antibacterial activities against vancomycin-resistant *Enterococci* and methicillin-resistant *Staphylococcus aureus* (MRSA).

Nitta *et al.* [203] isolated natural stilbenes (from the bark of *Shorea hemsleyana* and roots of *Cyphostemma bainessi*), which exhibited remarkable antibacterial activity against MRSA strain. Hemsleyanol D was one of the stilbenes tetramers mentioned in the previous study as the most active compound and had an inhibitory concentration of 2g/mL.

Famakin *et al.* [204] showed that combretastatin B5 (2',3',4-trihydroxyl-3,5,-'-trimethoxybibenzyl) has significant activity against *Staphylococcus aureus* with MIC of 16 g/ml but with lower activity towards *Pseudomonas aeruginosa* (125 g/ml), *Enterococcus faecalis* (125 g/ml) and slight activity against *Escherichia coli*.

ANTIVIRAL ACTIVITY OF FLAVONOID AND NON-FLAVONOID COMPOUNDS

Antiviral activity of flavonoids is divided based on their backbone structure into subclasses such as flavonols, flavanols, flavones, flavanones and other phenolics.

Antiviral Activity of Flavonols

Among flavonols, the antiviral effect of quercetin was the most extensively investigated. In cell cultures, quercetin revealed a dose-dependent antiviral action against HSV-1, HSV-2 (herpes-simplex-virus), poliovirus type 1 and respiratory syncytial virus [205, 206]. Quercetin was reported as an anti-HCV (hepatitis-c-virus) molecule and observed to have strong inhibitory activity on HCV production at 50 μM in cell culture [207]. Quercetin was reported to be active against influenza-A subtypes in *in-vivo* studies [208]. Current studies also mentioned the antiviral activity of quercetin against a wide spectrum of influenza virus strains [209].

Furthermore, quercetin and its derivatives were reported to be active against arthropod-borne mayaro virus, canine distemper virus, respiratory syndrome virus, porcine epidemic diarrhea virus and various other viruses [210 - 215]. There are numbers of other flavonols and their derivatives such as rutin, sulfated rutin, fisstin and myricetin are reported to be acting as antiviral compounds in different studies [216 - 219].

Kaempferol and kaempferol derivatives were also found to be active against human cytomegalovirus [220], HSV-1 and HSV-2 [221], have human immunodeficiency virus -1 inhibitory activity [222], influenza viruses [223, 224] and coronavirus [225].

Antiviral Activity of Flavones

The apigenin as a major compound from plant extracts was found to be active against HSV-1, poliovirus type 2, HCV [226, 227] and showed activity against adenoviruses (ADV) and hepatitis B virus in an *in-vitro* study [228].

Apigenin was found to be inhibiting African swine fever virus [229], suppressing viral IRES (internal ribosome entry site) activity [230, 231] and affects enterovirus-71 translation [232].

Apigenin and luteolin displayed highest inhibitory potencies of 7.9 μM and 4.3 μM (EC_{50} respectively) against HCV activity [233]. It was also reported that luteolin with an IC_{50} of 1.12 Mm, exhibited a functional inhibition of nonstructural protein-5B polymerase enzymatic function [234]. It was found that luteolin had an antiviral effect on HIV-1 reactivation [235] and showed significant inhibition of Epstein-Barr virus (EBV) reactivation in cells [236]. Xu *et al.* [237] found in the natural compounds based antiviral study, where the most potent inhibition was exhibited by luteolin through disruption of viral RNA replication among all 400 tested compounds.

Among flavones class, other compounds such as baicalein impaired avian influenza H5N1 virus replication [238], exerted anti-influenza activity [239] and proved as promising alternatives in the management of Tamiflu-resistant viruses [240]. It significantly reduced the protein levels of human cytomegalovirus [241, 242] and used for the treatment of early-stage infected HIV-1 cells [243].

Haid *et al.* [244] have isolated ladanein from *Marrubium peregrinum* L., with an anti-HCV activity at 2.5 μM concentration.

Antiviral Activity of Flavan-3-Ols

Among flavan-3-ols, the antiviral activity of tea compounds such as catechin and its derivatives epicatechin, EGC (epicatechin gallate) and EGCG are majorly investigated for antiviral activity [245]. EGCG was identified by different groups as a new inhibitor of HCV entry [246, 247]. In different studies, varied IC_{50} (5μM and 21μM) of EGCG was obtained and was also found to inhibit HCVpp entry in hepatoma-derived cells [246, 247].

EGCG has also been reported against herpes simplex virus, influenza virus [248 - 250] and as anti-HCV molecule [251]. EGCG could be used as a synergistic agent in combination with boceprevir or cyclosporin, with increased efficiency against HCV replication [252]. Furthermore, Nakayama *et al.* reported that EGCG could bind to the haemagglutinin of influenza virus [250] as well resulted in the inhibition of hemi fusion action between influenza virus and the cellular membrane [243]. According to Colpitts and Schang, EGCG by competing with sialic acid for binding to influenza A virus resulted in blocking the primary low-affinity attachment to cells [253].

Others have reported that EGCG has an antiviral effect against HIV infection [254, 255]. Additionally, Nakane and Ono showed that EGCG and ECG were effective at inhibiting HIV-1 reverse transcriptase [256, 257].

Furthermore, the green tea extracts showed inhibitory activity against HBV (Hepatitis B virus) [258]. EGCG is also reported to inhibit HBV replication by impairing HBV replicative intermediates of DNA synthesis [259].

Antiviral Activity of Flavanones

Naringenin belongs to the flavanones class and is reported to decrease the replication of a neurovirulent strain of sindbis virus *in vitro* [260] and also decreased sindbis and semliki forest virus-induced cytopathic effect [261]. The effect of naringenin was also studied on the secretion of HCV particles [262], which can block the assembly of intracellular HCV particles [263, 264]. After naringenin treatment at 200 μM concertation, the inhibitory activity was observed [262] in hepatocytes culture.

Hesperetin was found to exert the most potent anti-CHIKV (Chikungunya virus) effect with an IC_{50} of 8.5 µM during the virus intracellular replication [265]. Moreover, genistein was reported to inhibit HIV infection of resting CD4 T cells and macrophages [266]. It also inhibited the replication of HSV-1, HSV-2, by inhibiting the virus transcription [267, 268].

Antiviral Activity of other Phenolic Compounds

Silymarin and silibinin are flavonolignans of plant *Silybum marianum* and polyphenols of lignan and flavonoid moieties. Flavonolignans have been reported to have anti-HCV [269, 270], anti-inflammatory and immunomodulatory activity that could contribute to its hepatoprotective properties [271].

Besides this, several other dietary naturally occurring chlorogenic acids, phenolic acids and their derivatives were screened in one of our study for their inhibitory activity against neuraminidases (NAs) from *Clostridium perfringens*, H5N1 and recombinant H5N1 using a fluorometric assay [272]. In comparison to the established NA inhibitors oseltamivir and zanamivir, all tested compounds show increased NA inhibitory activity in a fluorometric assay. The caffeic acid derivatives seem promising compounds that suggested the use of plant material rich in chlorogenic acids as a treatment for viral infections.

CONCLUDING REMARKS

The 21st century faced major global healthcare problems due to the appearance and occurrence of multi-drug resistant microorganisms (MDR), which threaten the entire human life. Currently, after the ineffectiveness of traditional antibiotics, significant studies have been conducted on antimicrobial activities of medicinal plants secondary metabolites against MDR microorganisms. Over the past century, natural products are considered the major and promising sources of chemical diversity for starting materials of pharmaceutical drug discovery. In almost all therapeutic areas, many natural products or modified derivatives are successfully produced for treating various human diseases. Though, it is generally accepted that phytochemicals are less potent anti-infective than available anti-infective agents. However, future optimization of these compounds through structural modification may allow the development of biologically acceptable anti-infective agents. The isolated phenolic compounds of plants have been reported in general to possess various biological activities. The information collected in this review demonstrated the important uses of plants born phenolic compounds, which summarized the work done in the anti-infective research area. The *in-vitro* antimicrobial phenolic data published by various groups over the last decades has been briefly discussed.

Although increasing interest has encouraged more studies on the pharmacology of plant phenolics, however, there are still many areas for instance; systematic toxicity, and safety evaluation could be improved. Moreover, most of the antimicrobial activity studies have been carried out *in vitro*. Thus, the effectiveness of these compounds needs to be further investigated for their efficacy, safety, and bioavailability using *in vivo* assays, which will determine the real significance for the clinical use against pathogens.

CONFLICT OF INTEREST

The author declares that there is no conflict of interest in this chapter.

CONSENT FOR PUBLICATION

Not applicable.

ACKNOWLEDGEMENTS

Declared none.

REFERENCES

[1] Högberg LD, Heddini A, Cars O. The global need for effective antibiotics: challenges and recent advances. Trends Pharmacol Sci 2010; 31(11): 509-15. [http://dx.doi.org/10.1016/j.tips.2010.08.002] [PMID: 20843562]

[2] Laxminarayan R, Duse A, Wattal C, *et al.* Antibiotic resistance-the need for global solutions. Lancet Infect Dis 2013; 13(12): 1057-98. [http://dx.doi.org/10.1016/S1473-3099(13)70318-9] [PMID: 24252483]

[3] Jeu L, Piacenti FJ, Lyakhovetskiy AG, Fung HB. Voriconazole. Clin Ther 2003; 25(5): 1321-81. [http://dx.doi.org/10.1016/S0149-2918(03)80126-1] [PMID: 12867215]

[4] De Clercq E. New developments in anti-HIV chemotherapy. Curr Med Chem 2001; 8(13): 1543-72. [http://dx.doi.org/10.2174/0929867013371842] [PMID: 11562282]

[5] Poole K. Overcoming antimicrobial resistance by targeting resistance mechanisms. J Pharm Pharmacol 2001; 53(3): 283-94. [http://dx.doi.org/10.1211/0022357011775514] [PMID: 11291743]

[6] Taylor PW, Stapleton PD, Paul Luzio J. New ways to treat bacterial infections. Drug Discov Today 2002; 7(21): 1086-91. [http://dx.doi.org/10.1016/S1359-6446(02)02498-4] [PMID: 12546840]

[7] Kimberlin DW, Whitley RJ. Antiviral resistance: mechanisms, clinical significance, and future implications. J Antimicrob Chemother 1996; 37(3): 403-21. [http://dx.doi.org/10.1093/jac/37.3.403] [PMID: 9182098]

[8] Davies J. SECTION 3 The Advent of Modern Microbiology-In Praise of Antibiotics. ASM News-American Society for Microbiology 1999; 65: 304-10.

[9] Newman DJ, Cragg GM. Natural products as sources of new drugs over the last 25 years. J Nat Prod 2007; 70(3): 461-77.

[http://dx.doi.org/10.1021/np068054v] [PMID: 17309302]

[10] Wase NV, Wright PC. Systems biology of cyanobacterial secondary metabolite production and its role in drug discovery. Expert Opin Drug Discov 2008; 3(8): 903-29. [http://dx.doi.org/10.1517/17460441.3.8.903] [PMID: 23484967]

[11] Blunt JW, Copp BR, Munro MH, Northcote PT, Prinsep MR. Marine natural products. Nat Prod Rep 2005; 22(1): 15-61. [http://dx.doi.org/10.1039/b415080p] [PMID: 15692616]

[12] Kim H-S. Do not put too much value on conventional medicines. J Ethnopharmacol 2005; 100(1-2): 37-9. [http://dx.doi.org/10.1016/j.jep.2005.05.030] [PMID: 16039812]

[13] De Silva T. Industrial utilization of medicinal plants in developing countries. Medicinal plants for forest conservation and health care FAO, Rome 1997; 34-44.

[14] Butler MS. The role of natural product chemistry in drug discovery. J Nat Prod 2004; 67(12): 2141-53. [http://dx.doi.org/10.1021/np040106y] [PMID: 15620274]

[15] Clardy J, Walsh C. Lessons from natural molecules. Nature 2004; 432(7019): 829-37. [http://dx.doi.org/10.1038/nature03194] [PMID: 15602548]

[16] Fabricant DS, Farnsworth NR. The value of plants used in traditional medicine for drug discovery. Environ Health Perspect 2001; 109 (Suppl. 1): 69-75. [PMID: 11250806]

[17] Lewis WH, Elvin-Lewis MP. Medicinal plants as sources of new therapeutics. Ann Mo Bot Gard 1995; 16-24. [http://dx.doi.org/10.2307/2399976]

[18] Fraenkel GS. The raison d'ĕtre of secondary plant substances; these odd chemicals arose as a means of protecting plants from insects and now guide insects to food. Science 1959; 129(3361): 1466-70. [http://dx.doi.org/10.1126/science.129.3361.1466] [PMID: 13658975]

[19] Wink M. Evolution of secondary metabolites from an ecological and molecular phylogenetic perspective. Phytochemistry 2003; 64(1): 3-19. [http://dx.doi.org/10.1016/S0031-9422(03)00300-5] [PMID: 12946402]

[20] Stamp N. Out of the quagmire of plant defense hypotheses. Q Rev Biol 2003; 78(1): 23-55. [http://dx.doi.org/10.1086/367580] [PMID: 12661508]

[21] Tiwari S, Singh A. Toxic and sub-lethal effects of oleandrin on biochemical parameters of fresh water air breathing murrel, Channa punctatus. Bloch 2004.

[22] Lewis K, Ausubel FM. Prospects for plant-derived antibacterials. Nat Biotechnol 2006; 24(12): 1504-7. [http://dx.doi.org/10.1038/nbt1206-1504] [PMID: 17160050]

[23] Efferth T, Koch E. Complex interactions between phytochemicals. The multi-target therapeutic concept of phytotherapy. Curr Drug Targets 2011; 12(1): 122-32. [http://dx.doi.org/10.2174/138945011793591626] [PMID: 20735354]

[24] Farnsworth NR, Akerele O, Bingel AS, Soejarto DD, Guo Z. Medicinal plants in therapy. Bull World Health Organ 1985; 63(6): 965-81. [PMID: 3879679]

[25] McChesney JD, Venkataraman SK, Henri JT. Plant natural products: back to the future or into extinction. Phytochemistry 2007; 68(14): 2015-22. [http://dx.doi.org/10.1016/j.phytochem.2007.04.032] [PMID: 17574638]

[26] Braga LC, Leite AA, Xavier KG, *et al.* Synergic interaction between pomegranate extract and antibiotics against *Staphylococcus aureus*. Can J Microbiol 2005; 51(7): 541-7. [http://dx.doi.org/10.1139/w05-022] [PMID: 16175202]

[27] Adwan G, Mhanna M. Synergistic effects of plant extracts and antibiotics on *Staphylococcus aureus* strains isolated from clinical specimens. Middle East J Sci Res 2008; 3: 134-9.

[28] Pawlowska AM, Camangi F, Bader A, Braca A. Flavonoids of Zizyphus jujuba L. and Zizyphus spina-christi (L.) Willd (Rhamnaceae) fruits. Food Chem 2009; 112: 858-62. [http://dx.doi.org/10.1016/j.foodchem.2008.06.053]

[29] Halbwirth H. The creation and physiological relevance of divergent hydroxylation patterns in the flavonoid pathway. Int J Mol Sci 2010; 11(2): 595-621. [http://dx.doi.org/10.3390/ijms11020595] [PMID: 20386656]

[30] Naczk M, Shahidi F. Extraction and analysis of phenolics in food. J Chromatogr A 2004; 1054(1-2): 95-111. [http://dx.doi.org/10.1016/S0021-9673(04)01409-8] [PMID: 15553136]

[31] Scalbert A, Williamson G. Dietary intake and bioavailability of polyphenols. J Nutr 2000; 130(8S) (Suppl.): 2073S-85S. [http://dx.doi.org/10.1093/jn/130.8.2073S] [PMID: 10917926]

[32] Kang NJ, Shin SH, Lee HJ, Lee KW. Polyphenols as small molecular inhibitors of signaling cascades in carcinogenesis. Pharmacol Ther 2011; 130(3): 310-24. [http://dx.doi.org/10.1016/j.pharmthera.2011.02.004] [PMID: 21356239]

[33] Kim D-O, Lee KW, Lee HJ, Lee CY. Vitamin C equivalent antioxidant capacity (VCEAC) of phenolic phytochemicals. J Agric Food Chem 2002; 50(13): 3713-7. [http://dx.doi.org/10.1021/jf020071c] [PMID: 12059148]

[34] Eberhardt MV, Lee CY, Liu RH. Antioxidant activity of fresh apples. Nature 2000; 405(6789): 903-4. [http://dx.doi.org/10.1038/35016151] [PMID: 10879522]

[35] Korycka-Dahl MB, Richardson T, Foote CS. Activated oxygen species and oxidation of food constituents. CRC Crit Rev Food Sci Nutr 1978; 10(3): 209-41. [http://dx.doi.org/10.1080/10408397809527250] [PMID: 215383]

[36] Lavelli V, Hippeli S, Peri C, Elstner EF. Evaluation of radical scavenging activity of fresh and air-dried tomatoes by three model reactions. J Agric Food Chem 1999; 47(9): 3826-31. [http://dx.doi.org/10.1021/jf981372i] [PMID: 10552729]

[37] Rezk A, Nolzen J, Schepker H, Albach DC, Brix K, Ullrich MS. Phylogenetic spectrum and analysis of antibacterial activities of leaf extracts from plants of the genus Rhododendron. BMC Complement Altern Med 2015; 15: 67. [http://dx.doi.org/10.1186/s12906-015-0596-5] [PMID: 25879877]

[38] Shrestha A, Rezk A, Said IH, *et al.* Comparison of the polyphenolic profile and antibacterial activity of the leaves, fruits and flowers of Rhododendron ambiguum and Rhododendron cinnabarinum. BMC Res Notes 2017; 10(1): 297. [http://dx.doi.org/10.1186/s13104-017-2601-1] [PMID: 28728600]

[39] Hakeem Said I, Rezk A, Hussain I, *et al.* Metabolome Comparison of Bioactive and Inactive Rhododendron Extracts and Identification of an Antibacterial Cannabinoid(s) from Rhododendron collettianum. Phytochem Anal 2017; 28(5): 454-64. [http://dx.doi.org/10.1002/pca.2694] [PMID: 28612345]

[40] Grimbs A, Shrestha A, Rezk ASD, *et al.* Bioactivity in Rhododendron: A systemic analysis of antimicrobial and cytotoxic activities and their phylogenetic and phytochemical origins. Front Plant Sci 2017; 8: 551. [http://dx.doi.org/10.3389/fpls.2017.00551] [PMID: 28450876]

[41] Cowan MM. Plant products as antimicrobial agents. Clin Microbiol Rev 1999; 12(4): 564-82. [http://dx.doi.org/10.1128/CMR.12.4.564] [PMID: 10515903]

[42] Bomser JA, Singletary KW, Wallig MA, Smith MA. Inhibition of TPA-induced tumor promotion in

CD-1 mouse epidermis by a polyphenolic fraction from grape seeds. Cancer Lett 1999; 135(2): 151-7. [http://dx.doi.org/10.1016/S0304-3835(98)00289-4] [PMID: 10096423]

[43] Preuss HG, Montamarry S, Echard B, Scheckenbach R, Bagchi D. Long-term effects of chromium, grape seed extract, and zinc on various metabolic parameters of rats. Mol Cell Biochem 2001; 223(1-2): 95-102. [http://dx.doi.org/10.1023/A:1017961029492] [PMID: 11681727]

[44] He J, Chen Y, Farzan M, *et al.* CCR3 and CCR5 are co-receptors for HIV-1 infection of microglia. Nature 1997; 385(6617): 645-9. [http://dx.doi.org/10.1038/385645a0] [PMID: 9024664]

[45] Lotito SB, Frei B. Consumption of flavonoid-rich foods and increased plasma antioxidant capacity in humans: cause, consequence, or epiphenomenon. Free Radic Biol Med 2006; 41(12): 1727-46. [http://dx.doi.org/10.1016/j.freeradbiomed.2006.04.033] [PMID: 17157175]

[46] Beecher GR. Overview of dietary flavonoids: nomenclature, occurrence and intake. J Nutr 2003; 133(10): 3248S-54S. [http://dx.doi.org/10.1093/jn/133.10.3248S] [PMID: 14519822]

[47] Del Rio D, Rodriguez-Mateos A, Spencer JP, Tognolini M, Borges G, Crozier A. Dietary (poly) phenolics in human health: structures, bioavailability, and evidence of protective effects against chronic diseases. Antioxidants & redox signaling 2013; 18: 92-1818.

[48] Haminiuk CW, Maciel GM, Plata-Oviedo MS, Peralta RM. Phenolic compounds in fruits - an overview. Int J Food Sci Technol 2012; 47: 2023-44. [http://dx.doi.org/10.1111/j.1365-2621.2012.03067.x]

[49] Reinli K, Block G. Phytoestrogen content of foods - a compendium of literature values. Nutr Cancer 1996; 26(2): 123-48. [http://dx.doi.org/10.1080/01635589609514470] [PMID: 8875551]

[50] Rouseff RL, Martin SF, Youtsey CO. Quantitative survey of narirutin, naringin, hesperidin, and neohesperidin in citrus. J Agric Food Chem 1987; 35: 1027-30. [http://dx.doi.org/10.1021/jf00078a040]

[51] Hertog MG, Hollman PC, Katan MB. Content of potentially anticarcinogenic flavonoids of 28 vegetables and 9 fruits commonly consumed in the Netherlands. J Agric Food Chem 1992; 40: 2379-83. [http://dx.doi.org/10.1021/jf00024a011]

[52] Lee M-J, Wang Z-Y, Li H, *et al.* Analysis of plasma and urinary tea polyphenols in human subjects. Cancer Epidemiol Biomarkers Prev 1995; 4(4): 393-9. [PMID: 7655336]

[53] Santos-Buelga C, Scalbert A. Proanthocyanidins and tannin-like compounds - nature, occurrence, dietary intake and effects on nutrition and health. J Sci Food Agric 2000; 80: 1094-117. [http://dx.doi.org/10.1002/(SICI)1097-0010(20000515)80:7<1094::AID-JSFA569>3.0.CO;2-1]

[54] Moroney MA, Alcaraz MJ, Forder RA, Carey F, Hoult JR. Selectivity of neutrophil 5-lipoxygenase and cyclo-oxygenase inhibition by an anti-inflammatory flavonoid glycoside and related aglycone flavonoids. J Pharm Pharmacol 1988; 40(11): 787-92. [http://dx.doi.org/10.1111/j.2042-7158.1988.tb05173.x] [PMID: 2907559]

[55] Vlaskovska M, Drenska D, Ovcharov R. Effect of antioxidants, alone and in combination, on the inflammatory process. Probl Vutr Med 1990; 18: 19.

[56] Bors W, Saran M. Radical scavenging by flavonoid antioxidants. Free Radic Res Commun 1987; 2(4-6): 289-94. [http://dx.doi.org/10.3109/10715768709065294] [PMID: 3504810]

[57] Kroon PA, Faulds CB, Ryden P, Robertson JA, Williamson G. Release of covalently bound ferulic acid from fiber in the human colon. J Agric Food Chem 1997; 45: 661-7.

[http://dx.doi.org/10.1021/jf9604403]

[58] Clifford MN. Chlorogenic acids and other cinnamates - nature, occurrence and dietary burden. J Sci Food Agric 1999; 79: 362-72. [http://dx.doi.org/10.1002/(SICI)1097-0010(19990301)79:3<362::AID-JSFA256>3.0.CO;2-D]

[59] Lou Z, Wang H, Zhu S, Ma C, Wang Z. Antibacterial activity and mechanism of action of chlorogenic acid. J Food Sci 2011; 76(6): M398-403. [http://dx.doi.org/10.1111/j.1750-3841.2011.02213.x] [PMID: 22417510]

[60] Xie Y, Huang B, Yu K, Shi F, Liu T, Xu W. Caffeic acid derivatives: a new type of influenza neuraminidase inhibitors. Bioorg Med Chem Lett 2013; 23(12): 3556-60. [http://dx.doi.org/10.1016/j.bmcl.2013.04.033] [PMID: 23664211]

[61] Sung WS, Lee DG. Antifungal action of chlorogenic acid against pathogenic fungi, mediated by membrane disruption. Pure Appl Chem 2010; 82: 219-26. [http://dx.doi.org/10.1351/PAC-CON-09-01-08]

[62] Shin HS, Satsu H, Bae M-J, *et al.* Anti-inflammatory effect of chlorogenic acid on the IL-8 production in Caco-2 cells and the dextran sulphate sodium-induced colitis symptoms in C57BL/6 mice. Food Chem 2015; 168: 167-75. [http://dx.doi.org/10.1016/j.foodchem.2014.06.100] [PMID: 25172696]

[63] Han X, Shen T, Lou H. Dietary polyphenols and their biological significance. Int J Mol Sci 2007; 8: 950-88. [http://dx.doi.org/10.3390/i8090950]

[64] Schofield P, Mbugua D, Pell A. Analysis of condensed tannins: a review. Anim Feed Sci Technol 2001; 91: 21-40. [http://dx.doi.org/10.1016/S0377-8401(01)00228-0]

[65] Manach C, Scalbert A, Morand C, Rémésy C, Jiménez L. Polyphenols: food sources and bioavailability. Am J Clin Nutr 2004; 79(5): 727-47. [http://dx.doi.org/10.1093/ajcn/79.5.727] [PMID: 15113710]

[66] El Gharras H. Polyphenols: food sources, properties and applications - a review. Int J Food Sci Technol 2009; 44: 2512-8. [http://dx.doi.org/10.1111/j.1365-2621.2009.02077.x]

[67] Ignat I, Volf I, Popa VI. A critical review of methods for characterisation of polyphenolic compounds in fruits and vegetables. Food Chem 2011; 126(4): 1821-35. [http://dx.doi.org/10.1016/j.foodchem.2010.12.026] [PMID: 25213963]

[68] Côté J, Caillet S, Doyon G, Sylvain J-F, Lacroix M. Bioactive compounds in cranberries and their biological properties. Crit Rev Food Sci Nutr 2010; 50(7): 666-79. [http://dx.doi.org/10.1080/10408390903044107] [PMID: 20694928]

[69] Gescher K, Hensel A, Hafezi W, Derksen A, Kühn J. Oligomeric proanthocyanidins from Rumex acetosa L. inhibit the attachment of herpes simplex virus type-1. Antiviral Res 2011; 89(1): 9-18. [http://dx.doi.org/10.1016/j.antiviral.2010.10.007] [PMID: 21070811]

[70] Langcake P, Pryce RJ. A new class of phytoalexins from grapevines. Experientia 1977; 33(2): 151-2. [http://dx.doi.org/10.1007/BF02124034] [PMID: 844529]

[71] Bavaresco L, Fregoni C, Cantù E, Trevisan M. Stilbene compounds: from the grapevine to wine. Drugs Exp Clin Res 1999; 25(2-3): 57-63. [PMID: 10370866]

[72] Vitrac X, Bornet A, Vanderlinde R, *et al.* Determination of stilbenes (δ-viniferin, trans-astringin, trans-piceid, cis- and trans-resveratrol, ε-viniferin) in Brazilian wines. J Agric Food Chem 2005; 53(14): 5664-9. [http://dx.doi.org/10.1021/jf050122g] [PMID: 15998130]

[73] Paredes-López O, Cervantes-Ceja ML, Vigna-Pérez M, Hernández-Pérez T. Berries: improving human health and healthy aging, and promoting quality life-a review. Plant Foods Hum Nutr 2010; 65(3): 299-308.
[http://dx.doi.org/10.1007/s11130-010-0177-1] [PMID: 20645129]

[74] Morinaga N, Yahiro K, Noda M. Resveratrol, a natural polyphenolic compound, inhibits cholera toxin-induced cyclic AMP accumulation in Vero cells. Toxicon 2010; 56(1): 29-35.
[http://dx.doi.org/10.1016/j.toxicon.2010.03.009] [PMID: 20307562]

[75] Davin LB, Lewis NG. An historical perspective on lignan biosynthesis: monolignol, allylphenol and hydroxycinnamic acid coupling and downstream metabolism. Phytochem Rev 2003; 2: 257.
[http://dx.doi.org/10.1023/B:PHYT.0000046175.83729.b5]

[76] Saleem M, Kim HJ, Ali MS, Lee YS. An update on bioactive plant lignans. Nat Prod Rep 2005; 22(6): 696-716.
[http://dx.doi.org/10.1039/b514045p] [PMID: 16311631]

[77] Towers G, Stafford HA. Biochemistry of the mevalonic acid pathway to terpenoids In: Neil Towers GH, Helen A, Eds. Stafford. v 24Proceedings of the twenty-ninth Annual meeting of the Phytochemical Society of North America, held. June 16-20, 1989;
[http://dx.doi.org/10.1007/978-1-4684-8789-3]

[78] Schijlen EG, Ric de Vos CH, van Tunen AJ, Bovy AG. Modification of flavonoid biosynthesis in crop plants. Phytochemistry 2004; 65(19): 2631-48.
[http://dx.doi.org/10.1016/j.phytochem.2004.07.028] [PMID: 15464151]

[79] Tsao R. Chemistry and biochemistry of dietary polyphenols. Nutrients 2010; 2(12): 1231-46.
[http://dx.doi.org/10.3390/nu2121231] [PMID: 22254006]

[80] Crozier A, Jaganath IB, Clifford MN. Dietary phenolics: chemistry, bioavailability and effects on health. Nat Prod Rep 2009; 26(8): 1001-43.
[http://dx.doi.org/10.1039/b802662a] [PMID: 19636448]

[81] Day AJ, Rothwell JA, Morgan R. University of Leeds, Leeds, United Kingdom. Phytochemicals in health and disease 2004; 50

[82] Setchell KD, Brown NM, Lydeking-Olsen E. The clinical importance of the metabolite equol-a clue to the effectiveness of soy and its isoflavones. J Nutr 2002; 132(12): 3577-84.
[http://dx.doi.org/10.1093/jn/132.12.3577] [PMID: 12468591]

[83] Yuan JP, Wang JH, Liu X. Metabolism of dietary soy isoflavones to equol by human intestinal microflora-implications for health. Mol Nutr Food Res 2007; 51(7): 765-81.
[http://dx.doi.org/10.1002/mnfr.200600262] [PMID: 17579894]

[84] Ganry O. Phytoestrogen and breast cancer prevention. Eur J Cancer Prev 2002; 11(6): 519-22.
[http://dx.doi.org/10.1097/00008469-200212000-00002] [PMID: 12457102]

[85] Hollman PC, van Trijp JM, Buysman MN, *et al.* Relative bioavailability of the antioxidant flavonoid quercetin from various foods in man. FEBS Lett 1997; 418(1-2): 152-6.
[http://dx.doi.org/10.1016/S0014-5793(97)01367-7] [PMID: 9414116]

[86] Vijaya K, Ananthan S. Therapeutic efficacy of medicinal plants against experimentally induced shigellosis in guinea pigs. Indian J Pharm Sci 1996; 58: 191.

[87] Cushnie TP, Hamilton VE, Chapman DG, Taylor PW, Lamb AJ. Aggregation of *Staphylococcus aureus* following treatment with the antibacterial flavonol galangin. J Appl Microbiol 2007; 103(5): 1562-7.
[http://dx.doi.org/10.1111/j.1365-2672.2007.03393.x] [PMID: 17953567]

[88] Al-Saif SS, Abdel-Raouf N, El-Wazanani HA, Aref IA. Antibacterial substances from marine algae isolated from Jeddah coast of Red sea, Saudi Arabia. Saudi J Biol Sci 2014; 21(1): 57-64.
[http://dx.doi.org/10.1016/j.sjbs.2013.06.001] [PMID: 24596500]

[89] Hossion AM, Zamami Y, Kandahary RK, *et al.* Quercetin diacylglycoside analogues showing dual inhibition of DNA gyrase and topoisomerase IV as novel antibacterial agents. J Med Chem 2011; 54(11): 3686-703.
[http://dx.doi.org/10.1021/jm200010x] [PMID: 21534606]

[90] Lee K-A, Moon SH, Kim K-T, Mendonca AF, Paik H-D. Antimicrobial effects of various flavonoids on *Escherichia coli* O157: H7 cell growth and lipopolysaccharide production. Food Sci Biotechnol 2010; 19: 257-61.
[http://dx.doi.org/10.1007/s10068-010-0037-7]

[91] Liu H, Mou Y, Zhao J, *et al.* Flavonoids from Halostachys caspica and their antimicrobial and antioxidant activities. Molecules 2010; 15(11): 7933-45.
[http://dx.doi.org/10.3390/molecules15117933] [PMID: 21060300]

[92] ML Hossion A. Sasaki K. Novel quercetin glycosides as potent anti-MRSA and anti-VRE agents. Recent Patents Anti-Infect Drug Disc 2013; 8: 198-205.

[93] Ansari JA, Naz S, Tarar OM, Siddiqi R, Haider MS, Jamil K. Binding effect of proline-rich-proteins (PRPs) on *in vitro* antimicrobial activity of the flavonoids. Braz J Microbiol 2015; 46(1): 183-8.
[http://dx.doi.org/10.1590/S1517-838246120130280] [PMID: 26221106]

[94] Palacious P, Gutkind G, Randina R, De Torres R, Coussio J. Antimicrobial activity of B. crispa and B. notosergila. Genus Baccharis II. Planta Med 1983; 49: 128.
[PMID: 6657783]

[95] Mirzoeva OK, Grishanin RN, Calder PC. Antimicrobial action of propolis and some of its components: the effects on growth, membrane potential and motility of bacteria. Microbiol Res 1997; 152(3): 239-46.
[http://dx.doi.org/10.1016/S0944-5013(97)80034-1] [PMID: 9352659]

[96] Siriwong S, Thumanu K, Hengpratom T, Eumkeb G. Synergy and Mode of Action of Ceftazidime plus Quercetin or Luteolin on *Streptococcus pyogenes*. Evid Based Complement Alternat Med 2015; 2015759459
[http://dx.doi.org/10.1155/2015/759459] [PMID: 26576195]

[97] Alvesalo J, Vuorela H, Tammela P, Leinonen M, Saikku P, Vuorela P. Inhibitory effect of dietary phenolic compounds on *Chlamydia pneumoniae* in cell cultures. Biochem Pharmacol 2006; 71(6): 735-41.
[http://dx.doi.org/10.1016/j.bcp.2005.12.006] [PMID: 16414027]

[98] Rauha J-P, Remes S, Heinonen M, *et al.* Antimicrobial effects of Finnish plant extracts containing flavonoids and other phenolic compounds. Int J Food Microbiol 2000; 56(1): 3-12.
[http://dx.doi.org/10.1016/S0168-1605(00)00218-X] [PMID: 10857921]

[99] Basile A, Sorbo S, Giordano S, *et al.* Antibacterial and allelopathic activity of extract from *Castanea sativa* leaves. Fitoterapia 2000; 71 (Suppl. 1): S110-6.
[http://dx.doi.org/10.1016/S0367-326X(00)00185-4] [PMID: 10930721]

[100] Arima H, Danno G. Isolation of antimicrobial compounds from guava (Psidium guajava L.) and their structural elucidation. Biosci Biotechnol Biochem 2002; 66(8): 1727-30.
[http://dx.doi.org/10.1271/bbb.66.1727] [PMID: 12353635]

[101] el-Gammal AA, Mansour RM. Antimicrobial activities of some flavonoid compounds. Zentralbl Mikrobiol 1986; 141(7): 561-5.
[http://dx.doi.org/10.1016/S0232-4393(86)80010-5] [PMID: 3811648]

[102] Waage SK, Hedin PA. Quercetin 3-O-galactosyl-(1→ 6)-glucoside, a compound from narrowleaf vetch with antibacterial activity. Phytochemistry 1985; 24: 243-5.
[http://dx.doi.org/10.1016/S0031-9422(00)83528-1]

[103] Khanna P, Sharma O, Sehgal M, Bhargava C, Jain M, Goswami A, *et al.* Antimicrobial principles from tissue culture of some plant species. Indian J Pharm Sci 1980; 42: 113-7.

[104] Nishino C, Enoki N, Tawata S, Mori A, Kobayashi K, Fukushima M. Antibacterial activity of flavonoids against *Staphylococcus epidermidis*, a skin bacterium. Agric Biol Chem 1987; 51: 139-43. [http://dx.doi.org/10.1271/bbb1961.51.139]

[105] Pomilio AB, Buschi CA, Tomes CN, Viale AA. Antimicrobial constituents of Gomphrena martiana and Gomphrena boliviana. J Ethnopharmacol 1992; 36(2): 155-61. [http://dx.doi.org/10.1016/0378-8741(92)90016-K] [PMID: 1608273]

[106] Kuroyanagi M, Arakawa T, Hirayama Y, Hayashi T. Antibacterial and antiandrogen flavonoids from Sophora flavescens. J Nat Prod 1999; 62(12): 1595-9. [http://dx.doi.org/10.1021/np990051d] [PMID: 10654410]

[107] Simin K, Ali Z, Khaliq-Uz-Zaman SM, Ahmad VU. Structure and biological activity of a new rotenoid from Pongamia pinnata. Nat Prod Lett 2002; 16(5): 351-7. [http://dx.doi.org/10.1080/10575630290033114] [PMID: 12434992]

[108] Ng TB, Ling JM, Wang Z-T, Cai JN, Xu GJ. Examination of coumarins, flavonoids and polysaccharopeptide for antibacterial activity. Gen Pharmacol 1996; 27(7): 1237-40. [http://dx.doi.org/10.1016/0306-3623(95)02143-4] [PMID: 8981074]

[109] Faizi S, Ali M. Shamimin: a new flavonol C-glycoside from leaves of Bombax ceiba. Planta Med 1999; 65(4): 383-5. [http://dx.doi.org/10.1055/s-2006-960796] [PMID: 10364851]

[110] Liu H, Orjala J, Sticher O, Rali T. Acylated flavonol glycosides from leaves of Stenochlaena palustris. J Nat Prod 1999; 62(1): 70-5. [http://dx.doi.org/10.1021/np980179f] [PMID: 9917285]

[111] Yadava RN, Reddy KI. A new bio-active flavonol glycoside from the stems of Butea superba Roxb. J Asian Nat Prod Res 1998; 1(2): 139-45. [http://dx.doi.org/10.1080/10286029808039856] [PMID: 11261215]

[112] Cui Y, Oh YJ, Lim J, *et al.* AFM study of the differential inhibitory effects of the green tea polyphenol (-)-epigallocatechin-3-gallate (EGCG) against Gram-positive and Gram-negative bacteria. Food Microbiol 2012; 29(1): 80-7. [http://dx.doi.org/10.1016/j.fm.2011.08.019] [PMID: 22029921]

[113] Sudano Roccaro A, Blanco AR, Giuliano F, Rusciano D, Enea V. Epigallocatechin-gallate enhances the activity of tetracycline in staphylococci by inhibiting its efflux from bacterial cells. Antimicrob Agents Chemother 2004; 48(6): 1968-73. [http://dx.doi.org/10.1128/AAC.48.6.1968-1973.2004] [PMID: 15155186]

[114] Hisano M, Yamaguchi K, Inoue Y, *et al.* Inhibitory effect of catechin against the superantigen staphylococcal enterotoxin B (SEB). Arch Dermatol Res 2003; 295(5): 183-9. [http://dx.doi.org/10.1007/s00403-003-0411-x] [PMID: 12883826]

[115] Borris RP. Natural products research: perspectives from a major pharmaceutical company. J Ethnopharmacol 1996; 51(1-3): 29-38. [http://dx.doi.org/10.1016/0378-8741(95)01347-4] [PMID: 9213624]

[116] Sakanaka S, Shimura N, Aizawa M, Kim M, Yamamoto T. Preventive effect of green tea polyphenols against dental caries in conventional rats. Biosci Biotechnol Biochem 1992; 56(4): 592-4. [http://dx.doi.org/10.1271/bbb.56.592] [PMID: 27280653]

[117] Isogai E, Isogai H, Takeshi K, Nishikawa T. Protective effect of Japanese green tea extract on gnotobiotic mice infected with an *Escherichia coli* O157:H7 strain. Microbiol Immunol 1998; 42(2): 125-8. [http://dx.doi.org/10.1111/j.1348-0421.1998.tb02260.x] [PMID: 9572044]

[118] Ahn Y-J, Kawamura T, Kim M, Yamamoto T, Mitsuoka T. Tea polyphenols: selective growth inhibitors of Clostridium spp. Agric Biol Chem 1991; 55: 1425-6. [http://dx.doi.org/10.1080/00021369.1991.10870770]

[119] Radji M, Agustama RA, Elya B, Tjampakasari CR. Antimicrobial activity of green tea extract against isolates of methicillin-resistant *Staphylococcus aureus* and multi-drug resistant *Pseudomonas aeruginosa*. Asian Pac J Trop Biomed 2013; 3(8): 663-7. [http://dx.doi.org/10.1016/S2221-1691(13)60133-1] [PMID: 23905026]

[120] Cho Y-S, Schiller NL, Oh K-H. Antibacterial effects of green tea polyphenols on clinical isolates of methicillin-resistant *Staphylococcus aureus*. Curr Microbiol 2008; 57(6): 542-6. [http://dx.doi.org/10.1007/s00284-008-9239-0] [PMID: 18781360]

[121] Yi S, Wang W, Bai F, *et al.* Antimicrobial effect and membrane-active mechanism of tea polyphenols against *Serratia marcescens*. World J Microbiol Biotechnol 2014; 30(2): 451-60. [http://dx.doi.org/10.1007/s11274-013-1464-4] [PMID: 23979827]

[122] Yi SM, Zhu JL, Fu LL, Li JR. Tea polyphenols inhibit *Pseudomonas aeruginosa* through damage to the cell membrane. Int J Food Microbiol 2010; 144(1): 111-7. [http://dx.doi.org/10.1016/j.ijfoodmicro.2010.09.005] [PMID: 20884071]

[123] Jazani NH, Shahabi Sh, Ali AA. Antibacterial effects of water soluble green tea extracts on multi-antibiotic resistant isolates of *Pseudomonas aeruginosa*. Pak J Biol Sci 2007; 10(9): 1544-6. [http://dx.doi.org/10.3923/pjbs.2007.1544.1546] [PMID: 19069973]

[124] Mabe K, Yamada M, Oguni I, Takahashi T. *In vitro* and *in vivo* activities of tea catechins against *Helicobacter pylori*. Antimicrob Agents Chemother 1999; 43(7): 1788-91. [http://dx.doi.org/10.1128/AAC.43.7.1788] [PMID: 10390246]

[125] Ankolekar C, Johnson D, Pinto MdaS, Johnson K, Labbe R, Shetty K. Inhibitory potential of tea polyphenolics and influence of extraction time against *Helicobacter pylori* and lack of inhibition of beneficial lactic acid bacteria. J Med Food 2011; 14(11): 1321-9. [http://dx.doi.org/10.1089/jmf.2010.0237] [PMID: 21663484]

[126] Betts JW, Sharili AS, Phee LM, Wareham DW. *In vitro* activity of epigallocatechin gallate and quercetin alone and in combination *versus* clinical isolates of methicillin-resistant *Staphylococcus aureus*. J Nat Prod 2015; 78(8): 2145-8. [http://dx.doi.org/10.1021/acs.jnatprod.5b00471] [PMID: 26267658]

[127] Xu X, Zhou XD, Wu CD. The tea catechin epigallocatechin gallate suppresses cariogenic virulence factors of Streptococcus mutans. Antimicrob Agents Chemother 2011; 55(3): 1229-36. [http://dx.doi.org/10.1128/AAC.01016-10] [PMID: 21149622]

[128] Yoda Y, Hu Z-Q, Zhao WH, Shimamura T. Different susceptibilities of Staphylococcus and Gram-negative rods to epigallocatechin gallate. J Infect Chemother 2004; 10(1): 55-8. [http://dx.doi.org/10.1007/s10156-003-0284-0] [PMID: 14991521]

[129] Lee P, Tan KS. Effects of Epigallocatechin gallate against *Enterococcus faecalis*biofilm and virulence. Arch Oral Biol 2015; 60(3): 393-9. [http://dx.doi.org/10.1016/j.archoralbio.2014.11.014] [PMID: 25526623]

[130] Hull Vance S, Tucci M, Benghuzzi H. Evaluation of the antimicrobial efficacy of green tea extract (egcg) against *streptococcus pyogenesin vitro* - biomed 2011. Biomed Sci Instrum 2011; 47: 177-82. [PMID: 21525617]

[131] Sakanaka S, Juneja LR, Taniguchi M. Antimicrobial effects of green tea polyphenols on thermophilic spore-forming bacteria. J Biosci Bioeng 2000; 90(1): 81-5. [http://dx.doi.org/10.1016/S1389-1723(00)80038-9] [PMID: 16232822]

[132] Lee K-M, Kim W-S, Lim J, *et al.* Antipathogenic properties of green tea polyphenol epigallocatechin gallate at concentrations below the MIC against enterohemorrhagic *Escherichia coli* O157:H7. J Food Prot 2009; 72(2): 325-31. [http://dx.doi.org/10.4315/0362-028X-72.2.325] [PMID: 19350976]

[133] Yanagawa Y, Yamamoto Y, Hara Y, Shimamura T. A combination effect of epigallocatechin gallate, a major compound of green tea catechins, with antibiotics on *Helicobacter pylori* growth *in vitro*.

Current microbiology 2003; 47: 0244-49.

[134] Lee JH, Shim JS, Chung MS, Lim ST, Kim KH. *In vitro* anti-adhesive activity of green tea extract against pathogen adhesion. Phytother Res 2009; 23(4): 460-6. [http://dx.doi.org/10.1002/ptr.2609] [PMID: 19107860]

[135] Jeon J, Kim JH, Lee CK, Oh CH, Song HJ. The antimicrobial activity of (-)-epigallocatehin-3-gallate and green tea extracts against *Pseudomonas aeruginosa* and *Escherichia coli* isolated from skin wounds. Ann Dermatol 2014; 26(5): 564-9. [http://dx.doi.org/10.5021/ad.2014.26.5.564] [PMID: 25324647]

[136] Cho Y-S, Oh JJ, Oh K-H. Synergistic anti-bacterial and proteomic effects of epigallocatechin gallate on clinical isolates of imipenem-resistant Klebsiella pneumoniae. Phytomedicine 2011; 18(11): 941-6. [http://dx.doi.org/10.1016/j.phymed.2011.03.012] [PMID: 21596543]

[137] Yam TS, Hamilton-Miller JM, Shah S. The effect of a component of tea (Camellia sinensis) on methicillin resistance, PBP2′ synthesis, and beta-lactamase production in *Staphylococcus aureus*. J Antimicrob Chemother 1998; 42(2): 211-6. [http://dx.doi.org/10.1093/jac/42.2.211] [PMID: 9738838]

[138] Stapleton PD, Shah S, Anderson JC, Hara Y, Hamilton-Miller JM, Taylor PW. Modulation of β-lactam resistance in *Staphylococcus aureus* by catechins and gallates. Int J Antimicrob Agents 2004; 23(5): 462-7. [http://dx.doi.org/10.1016/j.ijantimicag.2003.09.027] [PMID: 15120724]

[139] Shiota S, Shimizu M, Mizushima T, *et al.* Marked reduction in the minimum inhibitory concentration (MIC) of β-lactams in methicillin-resistant *Staphylococcus aureus* produced by epicatechin gallate, an ingredient of green tea (Camellia sinensis). Biol Pharm Bull 1999; 22(12): 1388-90. [http://dx.doi.org/10.1248/bpb.22.1388] [PMID: 10746177]

[140] Tsuchiya H, Sato M, Miyazaki T, *et al.* Comparative study on the antibacterial activity of phytochemical flavanones against methicillin-resistant *Staphylococcus aureus*. J Ethnopharmacol 1996; 50(1): 27-34. [http://dx.doi.org/10.1016/0378-8741(96)85514-0] [PMID: 8778504]

[141] Wächter GA, Hoffmann JJ, Furbacher T, Blake ME, Timmermann BN. Antibacterial and antifungal flavanones from Eysenhardtia texana. Phytochemistry 1999; 52(8): 1469-71. [http://dx.doi.org/10.1016/S0031-9422(99)00221-6] [PMID: 10647219]

[142] Chacha M, Bojase-Moleta G, Majinda RR. Antimicrobial and radical scavenging flavonoids from the stem wood of Erythrina latissima. Phytochemistry 2005; 66(1): 99-104. [http://dx.doi.org/10.1016/j.phytochem.2004.10.013] [PMID: 15649516]

[143] Biyiti L, Pesando D, Puiseux-Dao S. Antimicrobial activity of two flavanones isolated from the Cameroonian plant Erythrina sigmoidea. Planta Med 1988; 54(2): 126-8. [http://dx.doi.org/10.1055/s-2006-962368] [PMID: 3406170]

[144] Deng Y, Lee JP, Tianasoa-Ramamonjy M, *et al.* New antimicrobial flavanones from Physena madagascariensis. J Nat Prod 2000; 63(8): 1082-9. [http://dx.doi.org/10.1021/np000054m] [PMID: 10978202]

[145] Tombola F, Campello S, De Luca L, *et al.* Plant polyphenols inhibit VacA, a toxin secreted by the gastric pathogen *Helicobacter pylori*. FEBS Lett 2003; 543(1-3): 184-9. [http://dx.doi.org/10.1016/S0014-5793(03)00443-5] [PMID: 12753930]

[146] Mandalari G, Bennett RN, Bisignano G, *et al.* Antimicrobial activity of flavonoids extracted from bergamot (Citrus bergamia Risso) peel, a byproduct of the essential oil industry. J Appl Microbiol 2007; 103(6): 2056-64. [http://dx.doi.org/10.1111/j.1365-2672.2007.03456.x] [PMID: 18045389]

[147] Fukai T, Marumo A, Kaitou K, Kanda T, Terada S, Nomura T. Anti-*Helicobacter pylori* flavonoids from licorice extract. Life Sci 2002; 71(12): 1449-63.

[http://dx.doi.org/10.1016/S0024-3205(02)01864-7] [PMID: 12127165]

[148] Burger O, Weiss E, Sharon N, Tabak M, Neeman I, Ofek I. Inhibition of *Helicobacter pylori* adhesion to human gastric mucus by a high-molecular-weight constituent of cranberry juice. Crit Rev Food Sci Nutr 2002; 42(3) (Suppl.): 279-84. [http://dx.doi.org/10.1080/10408390209351916] [PMID: 12058986]

[149] Vikram A, Jesudhasan PR, Jayaprakasha GK, Pillai SD, Jayaraman A, Patil BS. Citrus flavonoid represses Salmonella pathogenicity island 1 and motility in S. Typhimurium LT2. Int J Food Microbiol 2011; 145(1): 28-36. [http://dx.doi.org/10.1016/j.ijfoodmicro.2010.11.013] [PMID: 21168230]

[150] Vandeputte OM, Kiendrebeogo M, Rasamiravaka T, *et al.* The flavanone naringenin reduces the production of quorum sensing-controlled virulence factors in *Pseudomonas aeruginosa* PAO1. Microbiology (Reading) 2011; 157(Pt 7): 2120-32. [http://dx.doi.org/10.1099/mic.0.049338-0] [PMID: 21546585]

[151] Bakar NS, Zin NM, Basri DF. Synergy of flavone with vancomycin and oxacillin against vancomycin-intermediate Staphyloccus aureus. Pak J Pharm Sci 2012; 25(3): 633-8. [PMID: 22713953]

[152] Abuelsaad AS, Mohamed I, Allam G, Al-Solumani AA. Antimicrobial and immunomodulating activities of hesperidin and ellagic acid against diarrheic Aeromonas hydrophila in a murine model. Life Sci 2013; 93(20): 714-22. [http://dx.doi.org/10.1016/j.lfs.2013.09.019] [PMID: 24090709]

[153] Bae E-A, Han MJ, Kim D-H. *In vitro* anti-*Helicobacter pylori* activity of some flavonoids and their metabolites. Planta Med 1999; 65(5): 442-3. [http://dx.doi.org/10.1055/s-2006-960805] [PMID: 10454900]

[154] Bashir A, Abdalla A, Wasfi I, Hassan E, Amiri M, Crabb T. Flavonoids of Limonium axillare 1994. [http://dx.doi.org/10.3109/13880209409083017]

[155] Sato Y, Suzaki S, Nishikawa T, Kihara M, Shibata H, Higuti T. Phytochemical flavones isolated from Scutellaria barbata and antibacterial activity against methicillin-resistant *Staphylococcus aureus*. J Ethnopharmacol 2000; 72(3): 483-8. [http://dx.doi.org/10.1016/S0378-8741(00)00265-8] [PMID: 10996290]

[156] Miski M, Ulubelen A, Johansson C, Mabry TJ. Antibacterial activity studies of flavonoids from Salvia palaestina. J Nat Prod 1983; 46(6): 874-5. [http://dx.doi.org/10.1021/np50030a007] [PMID: 6677714]

[157] Encarnacion R, Ochoa N, Anthoni U, Christophersen C, Nielsen PH. Two new flavones from Calliandra californica. J Nat Prod 1994; 57(9): 1307-9. [http://dx.doi.org/10.1021/np50111a023] [PMID: 7798967]

[158] Iniesta-Sanmartin E, Tomas-Barberan F, Guirado A, Tomas-Lorente F. Antibacterial flavonoids from Helichrysum picardii and H. italicum. Planta Med 1990; 56: 648-9. [http://dx.doi.org/10.1055/s-2006-961300]

[159] Sato M, Fujiwara S, Tsuchiya H, *et al.* Flavones with antibacterial activity against cariogenic bacteria. J Ethnopharmacol 1996; 54(2-3): 171-6. [http://dx.doi.org/10.1016/S0378-8741(96)01464-X] [PMID: 8953432]

[160] Alcaráz LE, Blanco SE, Puig ON, Tomás F, Ferretti FH. Antibacterial activity of flavonoids against methicillin-resistant *Staphylococcus aureus* strains. J Theor Biol 2000; 205(2): 231-40. [http://dx.doi.org/10.1006/jtbi.2000.2062] [PMID: 10873434]

[161] Liu R, Zhang H, Yuan M, *et al.* Synthesis and biological evaluation of apigenin derivatives as antibacterial and antiproliferative agents. Molecules 2013; 18(9): 11496-511. [http://dx.doi.org/10.3390/molecules180911496] [PMID: 24048283]

[162] Benmalek Y, Yahia OA, Belkebir A, Fardeau M-L. Anti-microbial and anti-oxidant activities of

Illicium verum, Crataegus oxyacantha ssp monogyna and Allium cepa red and white varieties. Bioengineered 2013; 4(4): 244-8.
[http://dx.doi.org/10.4161/bioe.24435] [PMID: 23579100]

[163] Eumkeb G, Siriwong S, Thumanu K. Synergistic activity of luteolin and amoxicillin combination against amoxicillin-resistant *Escherichia coli* and mode of action. J Photochem Photobiol B 2012; 117: 247-53.
[http://dx.doi.org/10.1016/j.jphotobiol.2012.10.006] [PMID: 23159507]

[164] Lv P-C, Li H-Q, Xue J-Y, Shi L, Zhu H-L. Synthesis and biological evaluation of novel luteolin derivatives as antibacterial agents. Eur J Med Chem 2009; 44(2): 908-14.
[http://dx.doi.org/10.1016/j.ejmech.2008.01.013] [PMID: 18313801]

[165] Kummee S, Intaraksa N. Antimicrobial activity of Desmos chinensis leaf and Maclura cochinchinensis wood extracts. Songklanakarin J Sci Technol 2008; 30(5): 635-9.

[166] Ooi LS, Wang H, He Z, Ooi VE. Antiviral activities of purified compounds from Youngia japonica (L.) DC (Asteraceae, Compositae). J Ethnopharmacol 2006; 106(2): 187-91.
[http://dx.doi.org/10.1016/j.jep.2005.12.028] [PMID: 16469463]

[167] Abd-Alla HI, Abu-Gabal NS, Hassan AZ, El-Safty MM, Shalaby NM. Antiviral activity of Aloe hijazensis against some haemagglutinating viruses infection and its phytoconstituents. Arch Pharm Res 2012; 35(8): 1347-54.
[http://dx.doi.org/10.1007/s12272-012-0804-5] [PMID: 22941477]

[168] Dastidar SG, Manna A, Kumar KA, *et al.* Studies on the antibacterial potentiality of isoflavones. Int J Antimicrob Agents 2004; 23(1): 99-102.
[http://dx.doi.org/10.1016/j.ijantimicag.2003.06.003] [PMID: 14732323]

[169] Chin Y-P, Tsui K-C, Chen M-C, Wang C-Y, Yang C-Y, Lin Y-L. Bactericidal activity of soymilk fermentation broth by *in vitro* and animal models. J Med Food 2012; 15(6): 520-6.
[http://dx.doi.org/10.1089/jmf.2011.1918] [PMID: 22468646]

[170] Hatano T, Shintani Y, Aga Y, Shiota S, Tsuchiya T, Yoshida T. Phenolic constituents of licorice. VIII. Structures of glicophenone and glicoisoflavanone, and effects of licorice phenolics on methicillin-resistant *Staphylococcus aureus*. Chem Pharm Bull (Tokyo) 2000; 48(9): 1286-92.
[http://dx.doi.org/10.1248/cpb.48.1286] [PMID: 10993226]

[171] Lakshmi P, Ganapaty S, Lakshminarayana K. Antimicrobial activity of the root extracts of T. pumila and T. tinctoria on clinical and phytopathogens. J Pharm Res 2009; 2: 1694-6.

[172] Hatano T, Kusuda M, Tsugawa M, Taniguchi S, Shiota S, Tsuchiya T, *et al.* Effects of natural polyphenols on methicillin-resistant Staphylococcus aureus in relation to their chemical and physical properties Phytochemistry Research Progress. Nova Science Publishers, Inc. 2008; pp. 31-47.

[173] Verdrengh M, Collins LV, Bergin P, Tarkowski A. Phytoestrogen genistein as an anti-staphylococcal agent. Microbes Infect 2004; 6(1): 86-92.
[http://dx.doi.org/10.1016/j.micinf.2003.10.005] [PMID: 14738897]

[174] Wen A, Delaquis P, Stanich K, Toivonen P. Antilisterial activity of selected phenolic acids. Food Microbiol 2003; 20: 305-11.
[http://dx.doi.org/10.1016/S0740-0020(02)00135-1]

[175] Herald P, Davidson P. Antibacterial activity of selected hydroxycinnamic acids. J Food Sci 1983; 48: 1378-9.
[http://dx.doi.org/10.1111/j.1365-2621.1983.tb09243.x]

[176] Muthuswamy S, Rupasinghe HV. Fruit phenolics as natural antimicrobial agents: Selective antimicrobial activity of catechin, chlorogenic acid and phloridzin. J Food Agric Environ 2007; 5: 81.

[177] Bajko E, Kalinowska M, Borowski P, Siergiejczyk L, Lewandowski W. 5-O-Caffeoylquinic acid: A spectroscopic study and biological screening for antimicrobial activity. Lebensm Wiss Technol 2016; 65: 471-9.

[http://dx.doi.org/10.1016/j.lwt.2015.08.024]

[178] Puupponen-Pimiä R, Nohynek L, Meier C, *et al.* Antimicrobial properties of phenolic compounds from berries. J Appl Microbiol 2001; 90(4): 494-507. [http://dx.doi.org/10.1046/j.1365-2672.2001.01271.x] [PMID: 11309059]

[179] Dogasaki C, Shindo T, Furuhata K, Fukuyama M. Identification of chemical structure of antibacterial components against Legionella pneumophila in a coffee beverage. Yakugaku Zasshi 2002; 122(7): 487-94. [http://dx.doi.org/10.1248/yakushi.122.487] [PMID: 12136645]

[180] Furuhata K, Dogasaki C, Hara M, Fukuyama M. Inactivation of Legionella pneumophila by phenol compounds contained in coffee. Journal of Antibacterial and Antifungal Agents 2002.

[181] Lipińska L, Klewicka E, Sójka M. The structure, occurrence and biological activity of ellagitannins: a general review. Acta Sci Pol Technol Aliment 2014; 13(3): 289-99. [http://dx.doi.org/10.17306/J.AFS.2014.3.7] [PMID: 24887944]

[182] Piwowarski JP, Granica S, Zwierzyńska M, *et al.* Role of human gut microbiota metabolism in the anti-inflammatory effect of traditionally used ellagitannin-rich plant materials. J Ethnopharmacol 2014; 155(1): 801-9. [http://dx.doi.org/10.1016/j.jep.2014.06.032] [PMID: 24969824]

[183] Leshem R, Maharshak I, Ben Jacob E, Ofek I, Kremer I. The effect of nondialyzable material (NDM) cranberry extract on formation of contact lens biofilm by *Staphylococcus epidermidis*. Invest Ophthalmol Vis Sci 2011; 52(7): 4929-34. [http://dx.doi.org/10.1167/iovs.10-5335] [PMID: 21467179]

[184] Tapiainen T, Jauhiainen H, Jaakola L, *et al.* Biofilm formation and virulence of uropathogenic *Escherichia coli* in urine after consumption of cranberry-lingonberry juice. Eur J Clin Microbiol Infect Dis 2012; 31(5): 655-62. [http://dx.doi.org/10.1007/s10096-011-1355-2] [PMID: 21822564]

[185] Koo H, Duarte S, Murata RM, *et al.* Influence of cranberry proanthocyanidins on formation of biofilms by Streptococcus mutans on saliva-coated apatitic surface and on dental caries development *in vivo*. Caries Res 2010; 44(2): 116-26. [http://dx.doi.org/10.1159/000296306] [PMID: 20234135]

[186] Ulrey RK, Barksdale SM, Zhou W, van Hoek ML. Cranberry proanthocyanidins have anti-biofilm properties against *Pseudomonas aeruginosa*. BMC Complement Altern Med 2014; 14: 499. [http://dx.doi.org/10.1186/1472-6882-14-499] [PMID: 25511463]

[187] Joshi SS, Howell AB, D'Souza DH. Cronobacter sakazakii reduction by blueberry proanthocyanidins. Food Microbiol 2014; 39: 127-31. [http://dx.doi.org/10.1016/j.fm.2013.11.002] [PMID: 24387862]

[188] Chatterjee A, Yasmin T, Bagchi D, Stohs SJ. Inhibition of *Helicobacter pyloriin vitro* by various berry extracts, with enhanced susceptibility to clarithromycin. Mol Cell Biochem 2004; 265(1-2): 19-26. [http://dx.doi.org/10.1023/B:MCBI.0000044310.92444.ec] [PMID: 15543930]

[189] Park YJ, Biswas R, Phillips RD, Chen J. Antibacterial activities of blueberry and muscadine phenolic extracts. J Food Sci 2011; 76(2): M101-5. [http://dx.doi.org/10.1111/j.1750-3841.2010.01974.x] [PMID: 21535771]

[190] Lacombe A, Wu VC, White J, Tadepalli S, Andre EE. The antimicrobial properties of the lowbush blueberry (*Vaccinium angustifolium*) fractional components against foodborne pathogens and the conservation of probiotic Lactobacillus rhamnosus. Food Microbiol 2012; 30(1): 124-31. [http://dx.doi.org/10.1016/j.fm.2011.10.006] [PMID: 22265292]

[191] Liu X-L, Hao Y-Q, Jin L, Xu Z-J, McAllister TA, Wang Y. Anti-*Escherichia coli* O157:H7 properties of purple prairie clover and sainfoin condensed tannins. Molecules 2013; 18(2): 2183-99. [http://dx.doi.org/10.3390/molecules18022183] [PMID: 23396143]

[192] Krauze-Baranowska M, Majdan M, Hałasa R, *et al.* The antimicrobial activity of fruits from some cultivar varieties of Rubus idaeus and Rubus occidentalis. Food Funct 2014; 5(10): 2536-41. [http://dx.doi.org/10.1039/C4FO00129J] [PMID: 25131001]

[193] Engels C, Schieber A, Gänzle MG. Inhibitory spectra and modes of antimicrobial action of gallotannins from mango kernels (*Mangifera indica* L.). Appl Environ Microbiol 2011; 77(7): 2215-23. [http://dx.doi.org/10.1128/AEM.02521-10] [PMID: 21317249]

[194] Bag A, Bhattacharyya SK, Chattopadhyay RR. Isolation and identification of a gallotannin 1,2,6-tri-O-galloyl-β-D-glucopyranose from hydroalcoholic extract of Terminalia chebula fruits effective against multidrug-resistant uropathogens. J Appl Microbiol 2013; 115(2): 390-7. [http://dx.doi.org/10.1111/jam.12256] [PMID: 23683054]

[195] Mohan J, Gandhi AA, Bhavya BC, *et al.* Caspase-2 triggers Bax-Bak-dependent and -independent cell death in colon cancer cells treated with resveratrol. J Biol Chem 2006; 281(26): 17599-611. [http://dx.doi.org/10.1074/jbc.M602641200] [PMID: 16617056]

[196] Atef M, Abdel Hamid SE, Abdel Ghani M. The influence of diethylstilboestrol on the antibacterial activity *in vitro* of some antibiotics. Zentralbl Veterinärmed A 1979; 26(9): 709-14. [http://dx.doi.org/10.1111/j.1439-0442.1979.tb01652.x] [PMID: 119381]

[197] Inamori Y, Ogawa M, Nishiguchi K, *et al.* Phytogrowth-inhibitory and antimicrobial activities of 3,4′-dihydroxy-α,β-diethylstilbene, the isomer of diethylstilbestrol. Chem Pharm Bull (Tokyo) 1991; 39(1): 218-20. [http://dx.doi.org/10.1248/cpb.39.218] [PMID: 2049805]

[198] Wyrzykiewicz E, Prukała W, Kedzia B. Synthesis and antimicrobial properties of *N*-substituted derivatives of (E)-alpha-(or gamma)-azastilbenols. Farmaco (Societa chimica italiana: 1989) 1994; 49: 31-127.

[199] Wyrzykiewicz E, Błaszczyk A, Kędzia B. Synthesis and antimicrobial activity of (E)-acetoxystilbenes and α,α′-dibromoacetoxybibenzyls. Farmaco 2000; 55(2): 151-7. [http://dx.doi.org/10.1016/S0014-827X(99)00127-5] [PMID: 10782388]

[200] Wang W-B, Lai H-C, Hsueh P-R, Chiou RY-Y, Lin S-B, Liaw S-J. Inhibition of swarming and virulence factor expression in *Proteus mirabilis* by resveratrol. J Med Microbiol 2006; 55(Pt 10): 1313-21. [http://dx.doi.org/10.1099/jmm.0.46661-0] [PMID: 17005777]

[201] Augustine N, Goel AK, Sivakumar KC, Kumar RA, Thomas S. Resveratrol-a potential inhibitor of biofilm formation in Vibrio cholerae. Phytomedicine 2014; 21(3): 286-9. [http://dx.doi.org/10.1016/j.phymed.2013.09.010] [PMID: 24182988]

[202] Sakagami Y, Sawabe A, Komemushi S, *et al.* Antibacterial activity of stilbene oligomers against vancomycin-resistant Enterococci (VRE) and methicillin-resistant *Staphylococcus aureus* (MRSA) and their synergism with antibiotics. Biocontrol Sci 2007; 12(1): 7-14. [http://dx.doi.org/10.4265/bio.12.7] [PMID: 17408003]

[203] Nitta T, Arai T, Takamatsu H, Inatomi Y, Murata H, Iinuma M, *et al.* Antibacterial activity of extracts prepared from tropical and subtropical plants on methicillin-resistant *Staphylococcus aureus*. J Health Sci 2002; 48: 273-6. [http://dx.doi.org/10.1248/jhs.48.273]

[204] Famakin J, Katerere D. Isolation of an antibacterial stilbene from *Combretum woodii* (Combretaceae) leaves. Afr J Biotechnol 2005; 4(10): 1167-71.

[205] Kang BK, Lee JS, Chon SK, *et al.* Development of self-microemulsifying drug delivery systems (SMEDDS) for oral bioavailability enhancement of simvastatin in beagle dogs. Int J Pharm 2004; 274(1-2): 65-73. [http://dx.doi.org/10.1016/j.ijpharm.2003.12.028] [PMID: 15072783]

[206] Lyu S-Y, Rhim J-Y, Park W-B. Antiherpetic activities of flavonoids against herpes simplex virus type 1 (HSV-1) and type 2 (HSV-2) *in vitro*. Arch Pharm Res 2005; 28(11): 1293-301. [http://dx.doi.org/10.1007/BF02978215] [PMID: 16350858]

[207] Gonzalez O, Fontanes V, Raychaudhuri S, *et al.* The heat shock protein inhibitor Quercetin attenuates hepatitis C virus production. Hepatology 2009; 50(6): 1756-64. [http://dx.doi.org/10.1002/hep.23232] [PMID: 19839005]

[208] Cho W-K, Weeratunga P, Lee B-H, *et al.* Epimedium koreanum Nakai displays broad spectrum of antiviral activity *in vitro* and *in vivo* by inducing cellular antiviral state. Viruses 2015; 7(1): 352-77. [http://dx.doi.org/10.3390/v7010352] [PMID: 25609307]

[209] Wu W, Li R, Li X, *et al.* Quercetin as an antiviral agent inhibits influenza A virus (IAV) entry. Viruses 2015; 8(1): 6. [http://dx.doi.org/10.3390/v8010006] [PMID: 26712783]

[210] Carvalho OV, Botelho CV, Ferreira CG, *et al. In vitro* inhibition of canine distemper virus by flavonoids and phenolic acids: implications of structural differences for antiviral design. Res Vet Sci 2013; 95(2): 717-24. [http://dx.doi.org/10.1016/j.rvsc.2013.04.013] [PMID: 23664014]

[211] Chiang LC, Chiang W, Liu MC, Lin CC. *In vitro* antiviral activities of Caesalpinia pulcherrima and its related flavonoids. J Antimicrob Chemother 2003; 52(2): 194-8. [http://dx.doi.org/10.1093/jac/dkg291] [PMID: 12837746]

[212] dos Santos AE, Kuster RM, Yamamoto KA, *et al.* Quercetin and quercetin 3-O-glycosides from Bauhinia longifolia (Bong.) Steud. show anti-Mayaro virus activity. Parasit Vectors 2014; 7: 130. [http://dx.doi.org/10.1186/1756-3305-7-130] [PMID: 24678592]

[213] Gao J, Xiao S, Liu X, *et al.* Inhibition of HSP70 reduces porcine reproductive and respiratory syndrome virus replication *in vitro*. BMC Microbiol 2014; 14: 64. [http://dx.doi.org/10.1186/1471-2180-14-64] [PMID: 24625230]

[214] Johari J, Kianmehr A, Mustafa MR, Abubakar S, Zandi K. Antiviral activity of baicalein and quercetin against the Japanese encephalitis virus. Int J Mol Sci 2012; 13(12): 16785-95. [http://dx.doi.org/10.3390/ijms131216785] [PMID: 23222683]

[215] Song JH, Shim JK, Choi HJ. Quercetin 7-rhamnoside reduces porcine epidemic diarrhea virus replication *via* independent pathway of viral induced reactive oxygen species. Virol J 2011; 8: 460. [http://dx.doi.org/10.1186/1743-422X-8-460] [PMID: 21967756]

[216] Tao J, Hu Q, Yang J, *et al. In vitro* anti-HIV and -HSV activity and safety of sodium rutin sulfate as a microbicide candidate. Antiviral Res 2007; 75(3): 227-33. [http://dx.doi.org/10.1016/j.antiviral.2007.03.008] [PMID: 17459492]

[217] Wang C, Wang P, Chen X, Wang W, Jin Y. Saururus chinensis (Lour.) Baill blocks enterovirus 71 infection by hijacking MEK1-ERK signaling pathway. Antiviral Res 2015; 119: 47-56. [http://dx.doi.org/10.1016/j.antiviral.2015.04.009] [PMID: 25912818]

[218] Lin Y-J, Chang Y-C, Hsiao N-W, *et al.* Fisetin and rutin as 3C protease inhibitors of enterovirus A71. J Virol Methods 2012; 182(1-2): 93-8. [http://dx.doi.org/10.1016/j.jviromet.2012.03.020] [PMID: 22465253]

[219] Yu M-S, Lee J, Lee JM, *et al.* Identification of myricetin and scutellarein as novel chemical inhibitors of the SARS coronavirus helicase, nsP13. Bioorg Med Chem Lett 2012; 22(12): 4049-54. [http://dx.doi.org/10.1016/j.bmcl.2012.04.081] [PMID: 22578462]

[220] Mitrocotsa D, Mitaku S, Axarlis S, Harvala C, Malamas M. Evaluation of the antiviral activity of kaempferol and its glycosides against human cytomegalovirus. Planta Med 2000; 66(4): 377-9. [http://dx.doi.org/10.1055/s-2000-8550] [PMID: 10865462]

[221] Yarmolinsky L, Huleihel M, Zaccai M, Ben-Shabat S. Potent antiviral flavone glycosides from Ficus

benjamina leaves. Fitoterapia 2012; 83(2): 362-7.
[http://dx.doi.org/10.1016/j.fitote.2011.11.014] [PMID: 22155188]

[222] Behbahani M, Sayedipour S, Pourazar A, Shanehsazzadeh M. *In vitro* anti-HIV-1 activities of kaempferol and kaempferol-7-O-glucoside isolated from Securigera securidaca. Res Pharm Sci 2014; 9(6): 463-9.
[PMID: 26339261]

[223] Jeong HJ, Ryu YB, Park S-J, *et al.* Neuraminidase inhibitory activities of flavonols isolated from Rhodiola rosea roots and their *in vitro* anti-influenza viral activities. Bioorg Med Chem 2009; 17(19): 6816-23.
[http://dx.doi.org/10.1016/j.bmc.2009.08.036] [PMID: 19729316]

[224] Ha S-Y, Youn H, Song C-S, *et al.* Antiviral effect of flavonol glycosides isolated from the leaf of Zanthoxylum piperitum on influenza virus. J Microbiol 2014; 52(4): 340-4.
[http://dx.doi.org/10.1007/s12275-014-4073-5] [PMID: 24682996]

[225] Schwarz S, Sauter D, Wang K, *et al.* Kaempferol derivatives as antiviral drugs against the 3a channel protein of coronavirus. Planta Med 2014; 80(2-3): 177-82.
[http://dx.doi.org/10.1055/s-0033-1360277] [PMID: 24458263]

[226] Manvar D, Mishra M, Kumar S, Pandey VN. Identification and evaluation of anti hepatitis C virus phytochemicals from Eclipta alba. J Ethnopharmacol 2012; 144(3): 545-54.
[http://dx.doi.org/10.1016/j.jep.2012.09.036] [PMID: 23026306]

[227] Visintini Jaime MF, Redko F, Muschietti LV, Campos RH, Martino VS, Cavallaro LV. *In vitro* antiviral activity of plant extracts from Asteraceae medicinal plants. Virol J 2013; 10: 245.
[http://dx.doi.org/10.1186/1743-422X-10-245] [PMID: 23890410]

[228] Chiang LC, Ng LT, Cheng PW, Chiang W, Lin CC. Antiviral activities of extracts and selected pure constituents of Ocimum basilicum. Clin Exp Pharmacol Physiol 2005; 32(10): 811-6.
[http://dx.doi.org/10.1111/j.1440-1681.2005.04270.x] [PMID: 16173941]

[229] Hakobyan A, Arabyan E, Avetisyan A, Abroyan L, Hakobyan L, Zakaryan H. Apigenin inhibits African swine fever virus infection *in vitro*. Arch Virol 2016; 161(12): 3445-53.
[http://dx.doi.org/10.1007/s00705-016-3061-y] [PMID: 27638776]

[230] Lv X, Qiu M, Chen D, Zheng N, Jin Y, Wu Z. Apigenin inhibits enterovirus 71 replication through suppressing viral IRES activity and modulating cellular JNK pathway. Antiviral Res 2014; 109: 30-41.
[http://dx.doi.org/10.1016/j.antiviral.2014.06.004] [PMID: 24971492]

[231] Qian S, Fan W, Qian P, *et al.* Apigenin restricts FMDV infection and inhibits viral IRES driven translational activity. Viruses 2015; 7(4): 1613-26.
[http://dx.doi.org/10.3390/v7041613] [PMID: 25835532]

[232] Zhang W, Qiao H, Lv Y, *et al.* Apigenin inhibits enterovirus-71 infection by disrupting viral RNA association with trans-acting factors. PLoS One 2014; 9(10)e110429
[http://dx.doi.org/10.1371/journal.pone.0110429] [PMID: 25330384]

[233] Liu M-M, Zhou L, He P-L, *et al.* Discovery of flavonoid derivatives as anti-HCV agents *via* pharmacophore search combining molecular docking strategy. Eur J Med Chem 2012; 52: 33-43.
[http://dx.doi.org/10.1016/j.ejmech.2012.03.002] [PMID: 22445328]

[234] Luo G, Hamatake RK, Mathis DM, *et al.* De novo initiation of RNA synthesis by the RNA-dependent RNA polymerase (NS5B) of hepatitis C virus. J Virol 2000; 74(2): 851-63.
[http://dx.doi.org/10.1128/JVI.74.2.851-863.2000] [PMID: 10623748]

[235] Mehla R, Bivalkar-Mehla S, Chauhan A. A flavonoid, luteolin, cripples HIV-1 by abrogation of tat function. PLoS One 2011; 6(11)e27915
[http://dx.doi.org/10.1371/journal.pone.0027915] [PMID: 22140483]

[236] Williamson G, Clifford MN. Colonic metabolites of berry polyphenols: the missing link to biological activity. Br J Nutr 2010; 104 (Suppl. 3): S48-66.

[http://dx.doi.org/10.1017/S0007114510003946] [PMID: 20955650]

[237] Xu L, Su W, Jin J, *et al.* Identification of luteolin as enterovirus 71 and coxsackievirus A16 inhibitors through reporter viruses and cell viability-based screening. Viruses 2014; 6(7): 2778-95. [http://dx.doi.org/10.3390/v6072778] [PMID: 25036464]

[238] Sithisarn P, Michaelis M, Schubert-Zsilavecz M, Cinatl J Jr. Differential antiviral and anti-inflammatory mechanisms of the flavonoids biochanin A and baicalein in H5N1 influenza A virus-infected cells. Antiviral Res 2013; 97(1): 41-8. [http://dx.doi.org/10.1016/j.antiviral.2012.10.004] [PMID: 23098745]

[239] Nayak MK, Agrawal AS, Bose S, *et al.* Antiviral activity of baicalin against influenza virus H1N1-pdm09 is due to modulation of NS1-mediated cellular innate immune responses. J Antimicrob Chemother 2014; 69(5): 1298-310. [http://dx.doi.org/10.1093/jac/dkt534] [PMID: 24458510]

[240] Chung S-T, Chien P-Y, Huang W-H, Yao C-W, Lee A-R. Synthesis and anti-influenza activities of novel baicalein analogs. Chem Pharm Bull (Tokyo) 2014; 62(5): 415-21. [http://dx.doi.org/10.1248/cpb.c13-00897] [PMID: 24572377]

[241] Cotin S, Calliste C-A, Mazeron M-C, *et al.* Eight flavonoids and their potential as inhibitors of human cytomegalovirus replication. Antiviral Res 2012; 96(2): 181-6. [http://dx.doi.org/10.1016/j.antiviral.2012.09.010] [PMID: 23000494]

[242] Evers DL, Chao C-F, Wang X, Zhang Z, Huong S-M, Huang E-S. Human cytomegalovirus-inhibitory flavonoids: studies on antiviral activity and mechanism of action. Antiviral Res 2005; 68(3): 124-34. [http://dx.doi.org/10.1016/j.antiviral.2005.08.002] [PMID: 16188329]

[243] Kim M, Kim S-Y, Lee HW, *et al.* Inhibition of influenza virus internalization by (-)-epigallocatech-n-3-gallate. Antiviral Res 2013; 100(2): 460-72. [http://dx.doi.org/10.1016/j.antiviral.2013.08.002] [PMID: 23954192]

[244] Haid S, Novodomská A, Gentzsch J, Grethe C, Geuenich S, Bankwitz D, *et al.* A plant-derived flavonoid inhibits entry of all HCV genotypes into human hepatocytes 2012. [http://dx.doi.org/10.1053/j.gastro.2012.03.036]

[245] Song JM, Seong BL. Tea catechins as a potential alternative anti-infectious agent. Expert Rev Anti Infect Ther 2007; 5(3): 497-506. [http://dx.doi.org/10.1586/14787210.5.3.497] [PMID: 17547513]

[246] Calland N, Albecka A, Belouzard S, *et al.* (-)-Epigallocatechin-3-gallate is a new inhibitor of hepatitis C virus entry. Hepatology 2012; 55(3): 720-9. [http://dx.doi.org/10.1002/hep.24803] [PMID: 22105803]

[247] Chen C, Qiu H, Gong J, *et al.* (-)-Epigallocatechin-3-gallate inhibits the replication cycle of hepatitis C virus. Arch Virol 2012; 157(7): 1301-12. [http://dx.doi.org/10.1007/s00705-012-1304-0] [PMID: 22491814]

[248] Isaacs CE, Wen GY, Xu W, *et al.* Epigallocatechin gallate inactivates clinical isolates of herpes simplex virus. Antimicrob Agents Chemother 2008; 52(3): 962-70. [http://dx.doi.org/10.1128/AAC.00825-07] [PMID: 18195068]

[249] Song J-M, Lee K-H, Seong B-L. Antiviral effect of catechins in green tea on influenza virus. Antiviral Res 2005; 68(2): 66-74. [http://dx.doi.org/10.1016/j.antiviral.2005.06.010] [PMID: 16137775]

[250] Nakayama M, Suzuki K, Toda M, Okubo S, Hara Y, Shimamura T. Inhibition of the infectivity of influenza virus by tea polyphenols. Antiviral Res 1993; 21(4): 289-99. [http://dx.doi.org/10.1016/0166-3542(93)90008-7] [PMID: 8215301]

[251] Fukazawa H, Suzuki T, Wakita T, Murakami Y. A cell-based, microplate colorimetric screen identifies 7,8-benzoflavone and green tea gallate catechins as inhibitors of the hepatitis C virus. Biol Pharm Bull 2012; 35(8): 1320-7.

[http://dx.doi.org/10.1248/bpb.b12-00251] [PMID: 22863932]

[252] Ciesek S, von Hahn T, Colpitts CC, *et al.* The green tea polyphenol, epigallocatechin-3-gallate, inhibits hepatitis C virus entry. Hepatology 2011; 54(6): 1947-55. [http://dx.doi.org/10.1002/hep.24610] [PMID: 21837753]

[253] Colpitts CC, Schang LM. A small molecule inhibits virion attachment to heparan sulfate- or sialic acid-containing glycans. J Virol 2014; 88(14): 7806-17. [http://dx.doi.org/10.1128/JVI.00896-14] [PMID: 24789779]

[254] Kawai K, Tsuno NH, Kitayama J, *et al.* Epigallocatechin gallate, the main component of tea polyphenol, binds to CD4 and interferes with gp120 binding. J Allergy Clin Immunol 2003; 112(5): 951-7. [http://dx.doi.org/10.1016/S0091-6749(03)02007-4] [PMID: 14610487]

[255] Williamson MP, McCormick TG, Nance CL, Shearer WT. Epigallocatechin gallate, the main polyphenol in green tea, binds to the T-cell receptor, CD4: Potential for HIV-1 therapy. J Allergy Clin Immunol 2006; 118(6): 1369-74. [http://dx.doi.org/10.1016/j.jaci.2006.08.016] [PMID: 17157668]

[256] Nakane H, Ono K, Eds. Differential inhibition of HIV-reverse transcriptase and various DNA and RNA polymerases by some catechin derivatives. Nucleic acids symposium series 1989; (21): 6-115.

[257] Nakane H, Ono K. Differential inhibitory effects of some catechin derivatives on the activities of human immunodeficiency virus reverse transcriptase and cellular deoxyribonucleic and ribonucleic acid polymerases. Biochemistry 1990; 29(11): 2841-5. [http://dx.doi.org/10.1021/bi00463a029] [PMID: 1693287]

[258] Xu J, Wang J, Deng F, Hu Z, Wang H. Green tea extract and its major component epigallocatechin gallate inhibits hepatitis B virus *in vitro*. Antiviral Res 2008; 78(3): 242-9. [http://dx.doi.org/10.1016/j.antiviral.2007.11.011] [PMID: 18313149]

[259] He W, Li L-X, Liao Q-J, Liu C-L, Chen X-L. Epigallocatechin gallate inhibits HBV DNA synthesis in a viral replication - inducible cell line. World J Gastroenterol 2011; 17(11): 1507-14. [http://dx.doi.org/10.3748/wjg.v17.i11.1507] [PMID: 21472112]

[260] Paredes A, Alzuru M, Mendez J, Rodríguez-Ortega M. Anti-Sindbis activity of flavanones hesperetin and naringenin. Biol Pharm Bull 2003; 26(1): 108-9. [http://dx.doi.org/10.1248/bpb.26.108] [PMID: 12520185]

[261] Pohjala L, Utt A, Varjak M, *et al.* Inhibitors of alphavirus entry and replication identified with a stable Chikungunya replicon cell line and virus-based assays. PLoS One 2011; 6(12)e28923 [http://dx.doi.org/10.1371/journal.pone.0028923] [PMID: 22205980]

[262] Nahmias Y, Goldwasser J, Casali M, *et al.* Apolipoprotein B-dependent hepatitis C virus secretion is inhibited by the grapefruit flavonoid naringenin. Hepatology 2008; 47(5): 1437-45. [http://dx.doi.org/10.1002/hep.22197] [PMID: 18393287]

[263] Goldwasser J, Cohen PY, Lin W, *et al.* Naringenin inhibits the assembly and long-term production of infectious hepatitis C virus particles through a PPAR-mediated mechanism. J Hepatol 2011; 55(5): 963-71. [http://dx.doi.org/10.1016/j.jhep.2011.02.011] [PMID: 21354229]

[264] Khachatoorian R, Arumugaswami V, Raychaudhuri S, *et al.* Divergent antiviral effects of bioflavonoids on the hepatitis C virus life cycle. Virology 2012; 433(2): 346-55. [http://dx.doi.org/10.1016/j.virol.2012.08.029] [PMID: 22975673]

[265] Ahmadi A, Hassandarvish P, Lani R, Yadollahi P, Jokar A, Bakar SA, *et al.* Inhibition of chikungunya virus replication by hesperetin and naringenin. RSC Advances 2016; 6: 69421-30. [http://dx.doi.org/10.1039/C6RA16640G]

[266] Guo J, Xu X, Rasheed TK, *et al.* Genistein interferes with SDF-1- and HIV-mediated actin dynamics and inhibits HIV infection of resting CD4 T cells. Retrovirology 2013; 10: 62.

[http://dx.doi.org/10.1186/1742-4690-10-62] [PMID: 23782904]

[267] Argenta DF, Silva IT, Bassani VL, Koester LS, Teixeira HF, Simões CM. Antiherpes evaluation of soybean isoflavonoids. Arch Virol 2015; 160(9): 2335-42. [http://dx.doi.org/10.1007/s00705-015-2514-z] [PMID: 26156104]

[268] Qian K, Gao AJ, Zhu MY, *et al.* Genistein inhibits the replication of avian leucosis virus subgroup J in DF-1 cells. Virus Res 2014; 192: 114-20. [http://dx.doi.org/10.1016/j.virusres.2014.08.016] [PMID: 25197039]

[269] Polyak SJ, Morishima C, Shuhart MC, Wang CC, Liu Y, Lee DYW. Inhibition of T-cell inflammatory cytokines, hepatocyte NF-kappaB signaling, and HCV infection by standardized Silymarin. Gastroenterology 2007; 132(5): 1925-36. [http://dx.doi.org/10.1053/j.gastro.2007.02.038] [PMID: 17484885]

[270] Polyak SJ, Morishima C, Lohmann V, *et al.* Identification of hepatoprotective flavonolignans from silymarin. Proc Natl Acad Sci USA 2010; 107(13): 5995-9. [http://dx.doi.org/10.1073/pnas.0914009107] [PMID: 20231449]

[271] Morishima C, Shuhart MC, Wang CC, Paschal DM, Apodaca MC, Liu Y, *et al.* Silymarin inhibits *in vitro* T-cell proliferation and cytokine production in hepatitis C virus infection. Gastroenterology 2010; 138: 81-671. e2.

[272] Gamaleldin Elsadig Karar M, Matei M-F, Jaiswal R, Illenberger S, Kuhnert N. Neuraminidase inhibition of Dietary chlorogenic acids and derivatives - potential antivirals from dietary sources. Food Funct 2016; 7(4): 2052-9. [http://dx.doi.org/10.1039/C5FO01412C] [PMID: 27010419]

[273] Ohemeng K, Schwender C, Fu K, Barrett J. DNA gyrase inhibitory and antibacterial activity of some flavones (1). Bioorg Med Chem Lett 1993; 3: 225-30. [http://dx.doi.org/10.1016/S0960-894X(01)80881-7]

[274] Al-Karablieh N, Weingart H, Ullrich MS. Genetic exchange of multidrug efflux pumps among two enterobacterial species with distinctive ecological Niches. Int J Mol Sci 2009; 10(2): 629-45. [http://dx.doi.org/10.3390/ijms10020629] [PMID: 19333425]

[275] Said IH, Shah RL, Ullrich MS, Kuhnert N. Quantification of microbial uptake of quercetin and its derivatives using an UHPLC-ESI-QTOF mass spectrometry assay. Food Funct 2016; 7(9): 4082-91. [http://dx.doi.org/10.1039/C6FO00652C] [PMID: 27711903]

[276] Serra DO, Mika F, Richter AM, Hengge R. The green tea polyphenol EGCG inhibits *E. coli* biofilm formation by impairing amyloid curli fibre assembly and downregulating the biofilm regulator CsgD *via* the σ(E) -dependent sRNA RybB. Mol Microbiol 2016; 101(1): 136-51. [http://dx.doi.org/10.1111/mmi.13379] [PMID: 26992034]

[277] Asahi Y, Noiri Y, Miura J, *et al.* Effects of the tea catechin epigallocatechin gallate on *Porphyromonas gingivalis* biofilms. J Appl Microbiol 2014; 116(5): 1164-71. [http://dx.doi.org/10.1111/jam.12458] [PMID: 24471579]

CHAPTER 3

Herbal Medicine in Russia's History: The Use of Herbal Medicine for Infectious Diseases in Russia's History

Mary Schaeffer Conroy[1,*]

[1] *Emeritus Professor, Department of History, University of Colorado, Denver, USA*

Abstract: The pandemic of COVID-19 is a grim reminder of the fact that viruses can be very contagious and that devising a vaccine and treatments against a viral disease is difficult and time-consuming. Our ancestors grappled with this problem for some infectious diseases until the late 19th century—and for others into the late 20th century. The chief weapons against infectious diseases were soap, disinfectants, isolation and quarantine, destruction of tainted items, and application of botanicals for symptoms of the viral diseases. This chapter describes Russians' multi-millennia experiences in treating infectious diseases with botanicals—from their earliest recorded history down to the present. The chapter is based on Russian-language sources—for the early period on information from chronicles and herbals recorded by Russian medical historians and for the modern period based on my personal research into pharmaceutical books and journal articles, interviews, and case records of practicing phytotherapists and healers.

Keywords: Anthrax, Botanical Research, Cholera, Epidemics, First World War, Herbals, Infectious Diseases, *Narodnaia Meditsina* Viruses, Post-Soviet Russia: Chronicles, Phytotherapy, Russia, Soviet Union, Smallpox, Second World War, Typhus, Typhoid.

INTRODUCTION

In this era of the new coronavirus, COVID-19, for which there is no vaccine, and no specific cure, it is advisable to look to the use of plants against infectious diseases in Russia. Herbal medicine has a long continuum in Russia. The use of botanicals to treat diseases and medical problems has been a key component of Russian medicine from the dawn of Russia's history in the 10th and 11th centuries of our era (A. D.) down through the 21st century, not only on the part of common people but also on the part of pharmacologists and medical specialists.

* **Corresponding author Mary Schaeffer Conroy:** Department of History, University of Colorado, Denver, United States; Tel: 13037616238; E-mail: maryesconroy@gmail.com

Ferid Murad, Atta-ur-Rahman, Ka Bian (Eds.)

Indeed, phytotherapy—the use of plants to treat medical problems and diseases--is not something new and trendy in present-day Russia as in the United States, where in recent decades the application of botanicals has been investigated as an alternative to the application of antibiotics, following findings that bacteria—particularly the frightening new "superbugs"-- are resistant to the antibiotics that have been liberally applied since the late 1940s. Rather, in addition to the application of vaccines and chemically synthesized medicines—the so-called "magic bullets" against infectious diseases—not only have Soviet citizens and émigrés from the Soviet Union continued to use popular medicine (*narodnaia meditsina*) and more specifically plants to treat diseases and medical problems, thus building up a huge reservoir of empirical evidence about the efficacy of medicinal botanicals, but pharmacologists, bio-chemists and medical personal have continued to publish research on the chemical formulae and application of botanicals in medicine until the present time. Unfortunately, since both the popular and the scholarly evidence on medicinal botanicals is in the Russian language, where as English has become the lingua franca of international science, few outsiders are conversant with Russian use of botanicals. The purpose of this chapter is to rectify that situation.

This chapter recounts the use of plants in Russia's history—particularly against infectious diseases—down to the present time for an English-speaking audience. The chapter follows a chronological format describing the use of medicinal botanicals against infectious diseases in the dim past down to the uses of phytotherapy at present for key infectious diseases, particularly COVID-19. Readers will see that occupying the vast Eurasian landmass, Russians were influenced by China and other oriental countries, by India, and by Middle Eastern peoples in their use of medicinal plants for infectious as well as chronic diseases. In the 18th and 19th centuries, familiarity with native medicinal botanicals led Russian medical specialists to repudiate bleeding and the harsh therapeutics that were fashionable in England and the United States at that time. In the 20th century, the use of medicinal botanicals was widespread in the Soviet Union, for reasons described in this chapter, resulting in less use of factory-produced antibiotics than in the United States and Western Europe. Phytotherapy continues to have a marked presence in post-Soviet Russia and the newly independent countries emerging from the collapsed Soviet Union. The use of popular medicine, and specifically medicinal botanicals, continues amongst émigrés from the Soviet Union living abroad, particularly those living in the United States.

HERBAL MEDICINES IN RUSSIAN HISTORY

Early Russia: Selected Use of Global Remedies in Health Care

It is theorized that the original home of the Slavic peoples was in central Europe—roughly in the area of modern-day Poland. Some Slavs moved into the territory later known as Russia by the 6th century A. D. The culture of these eastern Slavs, including their medical practices, was influenced by the vast Eurasian landmass in which they lived. Plants abounded—some of which were different from those in Western Europe. Additionally, the eastern Slavs traded with, fought against, and intermarried Finno-Ugric, Turkic, Iranian, and other peoples already residing in the landmass that stretched from Mongolia and China to the Mediterranean Sea.

From prehistoric times through the 13th and 14th centuries, migrant people continually moved from the east westward across the plains (or steppes) of Siberia and latter-day Russia/Ukraine to the Mediterranean Sea. Numerous waves of nomadic, horseback-riding peoples coursed across the steppes of Siberia in the first millennium before our era (B. C.) through the first millennium of our era, some moving into central Europe, even western Europe, and the Balkans. For Russia, the Mongols would be the last of these peoples, setting up their headquarters at the mouth of the Volga in the 13th century A. D. The Russian section of the Mongol Empire subsequently splintered into little khanates that lasted until Russians conquered them in the 16th, 17th and 18th centuries.

The Iranian and Turkic peoples living in Central Asia and eastern Siberia connected with China. They imported Chinese brides and their delicate carriages in the 6th century B. C. as the frozen graves of golden-clad rulers in the Altai mountains attest. Chinese medicine played a role in Russian medicine. Rhubarb, grown on the Chinese-Mongolian border was a major Russian export to Western Europe from the 17th through the early 19th centuries, as this chapter later discusses. The Mongol Doctor Peter Aleksandrovich Badmaev, an herbalist, who had studied Chinese and Tibetan medicine, practiced at the court of Tsar Nicholas II in the early 20th century, focusing on help for little Alexei, the hemophilic heir to the throne [1].

For medical, cultural, and political repercussions, equally important were the movements of Arabs northward up the Volga River into Russia and Central Asia and the migration of Scandinavians, in their shallow boats down the Volga River and the Dnieper River southward through Russia to the Bosporus.

First came the Arabs. The Caucasus itself was and still is home to a multitude of ethnic, linguistic, and religious groups. Muslim Arabs moved north through the Caucasus mountains and along the Volga River into Russia in the 8th century. Insofar as medicine and pharmacy were concerned, Arabs played a key role in both medieval Europe and Russia. Arabs who moved to Sicily, Italy, and Spain had preserved the medical lore and philosophy of the Greeks and Romans. This led to the establishment of a medical school in Salerno in the 9th century and medical schools in succeeding centuries in Montpellier, Naples, Padua, and

Bologna [2].

Arabic presence in Russia did not lead to the establishment of medical schools. However, the conversion of Iranian and Turkic peoples living in the steppes of Central Asia to Islam did influence medical care in those regions and also did so in Russia, situated west of the Ural Mountains. The Persian polymath Ibn Sina, (Avicenna), author of more than 450 works in 29 areas of science, including medicine and philosophy, lived in the ancient Central Asian cities of Bukhara and Khoresm [3]. His works were known to Russians and revered for centuries.

Shortly after the arrival of Arabs, Vikings mainly from Sweden moved into Russia. They intermarried with Slavic people, adopted the Slavic language, and became the first rulers of Russia. Russia from the 10th, 11th centuries down through the 15th century was a conglomerate of approximately ten principalities, ruled by hybrid Scandinavian-Slavic princes, and three city states, run by burghers.

The Norsemen were not so much interested in Russia but rather desired to trade with and possibly conquer Constantinople, the capital of the Byzantine Empire at that time. They thus linked the eastern Slavs to Byzantine and Greek culture [4]. Contacts with the Byzantine Empire influenced Russian culture and medical care. The eastern Slavs were converted to Christianity under the aegis of Bulgarian monks who brought them the Cyrillic alphabet, monasticism, the writing of chronicles, and elements of Byzantine art, architecture, and music. Russian monasteries established hospitals from the 11th century. Russian monks translated medical treatises from Greek and Latin into the Slavonic language. Doctors also came to Russia from Byzantium, Syria, Armenia, and Georgia. The monks and doctors were conversant with medicinal plants [5].

Medical practices from Western and Central Europe also entered Russia. The city-state of Novgorod, dominated by merchants with a hired prince to lead necessary armies, was a member of the Hanseatic League of German trading cities. From the 13th century through the 17th century, several western Russian and Ukrainian principalities were under the domination of Lithuania-Poland. The Russian princes regarded the militant Lithuanian princes as a counterweight to Mongols who had set up headquarters in the Volga delta in the 13th century and demanded tax payments and military conscripts. From the mid-13th century, “through a shrewd combination of warfare, dynastic marriages and diplomacy,” according to historian Walter G. Moss, Lithuanian prince Gedymin “spread Lithuanian control over...Belorussia and began penetrating southward into Ukraine.” [6] In 1386, a marriage between the daughter of the Polish King and a Lithuanian prince linked the two countries dynastically. In 1364, Polish King Casimir III “the Great” founded Jagiellonian University in Krakow, which was made famous by the astronomy discoveries of Copernicus. The university also had a medical faculty.

The Polish-Lithuanian Commonwealth continued to rule the territories now known as Belarus and Ukraine until the mid-17th century when Moscow, then ruled by the Romanov family, acquired eastern Ukraine up to the Dnieper River [7]. Tsarina Catherine the Great would acquire the western part of Ukraine and the western part of Belarus in the partitions of "Poland" in the second half of the 18th century [8].

Use of Herbs for Infectious Diseases in Early Russia

Our information about medical care in Russia in this early period is known from Law codes, from chronicles written in the principalities and city states, and from some 250 extant herbals. The first Russian Law code, *Russkaia Pravda*, issued by Prince Yaroslav "the Wise" in the early 11th century, and law codes issued by his sons later in the century, set forth money payments as punishments for murders and egregious crimes and payments to doctors in cases of maiming one's enemy [9].

The "*Shestodneve*" or Six Days Herbal described the application of medicinal botanicals to treat medical problems—specifically aconite, boligolova or *Conium* (family *Apiaceae)*, and belena (Hyoscyamus) [10]. Though all are poisonous, belena was used in Russian popular medicine into the 20th century to assuage pain from toothaches [11]. In the 12th century, the granddaughter of Prince Vladimir Monomakh, ruler of Kiev in modern-day Ukraine, compiled an herbal called, "Alimma" or "Salves" in which she described various diseases and treatments for them such as onions mixed with honey. In the city state of Novgorod, herbs were sold in the market. Many came from Egypt or were herbs not known in western Europe [12]. In 12th century Novgorod, the bark of the ash tree was used to treat the symptoms of malaria, which was endemic and sometimes epidemic in Russia through the 20th century. The bark of the ash tree had the same effect of quelling fever as did quinine—cinchona bark from south America not being available in Russia at that time [13]. The leaves of bagul'nik (Lédum, family *Ericaceae*) were used to treat the symptoms of tuberculosis.

Other medicinal herbs, citied in medieval Russian herbals but not used in Western Europe, include garlic, onion, the hemostatic, anti-inflammatory, and bactericide krapiva or nettles (*Urtica dioica L*), podorozhnik (*Plantago psyllium*, *Plantago major L.*), artemisia, shipovnik (*Rosa rogusa*), lipovei svet, valerian root, licorice root, juniper berries, birch leaves and sap, turpentine, vinegar—as well as arsenic, antimony, silver, and copper vitriol [14]. The plant items—particularly licorice, birch leaves, juniper berries, and *Rosa rogusa*—were still used in the 1970s to ward off and treat the symptoms of infectious diseases, including those caused by coronaviruses. For example, one form of podorozhnik--*Plantago psyllium*--was used to treat tumors, boils, inflammation of the eyes, and ailments of the stomach and digestive tract, as well as chronic colitis and gastritis. A second form of podorozhnik--*Plantago major L.*—contains vitamins A, C, and K and was used from ancient times to treat infectious diseases such as tuberculosis of the lungs, bronchitis and coughs, infections of the urinary tract, and boils [15]. Shipovnik or *Rosa rogusa* was still used in the 1970s to produce vitamin products—pills, teas, etc. (that could strengthen the immune system) and also to treat inflammation of the liver and urinary tract, and stomach ulcers—the latter now known to be caused by a bacterial infection [16]. Krapiva or nettles were used to treat wounds during the First World War [17]. Birch leaves (*Betula Verrucosa Ehrh*) were used to treat bronchitis as late as the 1980s [18]. Licorice root was used through the 20th century to treat respiratory problems from head colds (caused by one form of coronavirus) and was a major export from Russia to the United States, as is described further in this chapter [19].

Although there were no double-blind trials of the botanicals used in medieval Russia, the continuous use, over centuries, of similar plants to treat similar symptoms testifies to the efficacy of the botanicals.

Muscovite Russia: 14th century through the 17th century: Centralization and Globalization of Pharmacy

In the 15th century, the Prince of Moscow, Ivan III, began "gathering the Russian lands," that is, unifying the Russian principalities under Muscovite control. As a result, Russia was known to the world of that time as "Muscovy." This term continued to apply to Russia until the early 18th century. In the 16th century, the son of Ivan III and his grandson, Tsar Ivan IV, continued the process of bringing formerly independent principalities and city-states under the control of Moscow. Ivan IV fought Lithuania-Poland hoping to recover Russian territory that had passed under the control of the Lithuanian-Polish Commonwealth. He also fought Sweden, which ruled the southern literal of the Baltic Sea, for an outlet to that body of water. Ivan was not successful in these endeavors, but he did subordinate the Mongol khanates of Kazan, Astrakhan and Sibir' to allow Russian fur traders and explorers to expand across Siberia. He also organized trade with England, allowing the English to set up a depot on the Northern Dvina River and giving them access through the White Sea. Trade relations with Holland followed.

During this period of Muscovite expansion, foreign physicians and pharmacologists as well as other specialists were invited into Russia. Ivan III's second wife was Zoe or Sophia Paleologa--niece of the last Byzantine Emperor who fled Constantinople when it was conquered by the Ottoman Turks in May of 1453. From the age of five, Sophia had lived in Rome, as a ward of the Pope. After Ivan III married Sophia, Moscow was called "The Third Rome." To beautify the city, which became the capital of the Russian principalities Ivan brought under his control, he invited architects from Italy and Switzerland to build the famous "Faceted Palace" and churches in the Kremlin fortress, situated in Moscow's center [20]. A physician and pharmacist from Greece arrived in 1483 [21]. The Muscovite government now became an elaborate bureaucracy to collect taxes from the subordinate principalities and city states and generally administer them. Medicine and pharmacy were centralized in a government body called the Pharmacy Department (*Aptekarskii Prikaz*). A court pharmacy was established in 1581 by Tsar Theodore, son of Ivan IV. Of the foreign physicians and pharmacists (the two specialties being entwined at this time) the most famous was James Frencham but there were others as well. In the early 17th century, scions of the Romanov family—nobles from Kostroma, were elected to the throne of Russia. During the reigns of the first three Romanovs in the 17th century, a network of pharmacy warehouses and pharmacy gardens was established, in great part to supply the army. Additionally, a pharmacy for civilians also was opened in Moscow. A collection of wild medicinal plants was ordained [22].

Pandemics and Epidemics of Infectious Diseases in Russia: Herbal and Other Remedies

The English botanist James Tradescant was impressed with the herbals and knowledge of medicinal plants in Muscovite Russia [23]. In addition to the use of medicinal plants against infectious diseases on a small scale, as noted above, some botanicals were advocated during the epidemics and pandemics that occurred in Russia from the 14th through the 19th centuries. Plagues and pestilence were recorded in the chronicles of various early Russian principalities and city states as well in travelers' accounts. The Bubonic plague or the Black Death began in Central Asia but, strangely, circled around the globe before coming to Russian territory only in 1351 [24]. Medical historians hypothesize that bubonic--or pneumonic plague--was the disease described in the Russian manuscript "Ladoze" in 1352. Bubonic plague was mentioned again in 1424 in Karelia, in 1471 in Ustiug where it killed 12,000 people, and in 1669 in the Arctic Solovetskii Islands in the far north [25]. Medical historians also hypothesize that the pestilence among horses mentioned in 1571 in Ustiug referred to anthrax. Definite reference to anthrax was made by Dr. S. A. Andrievskii in 1788-1789 in Siberia—hence the name "Siberian plague". [26] An infectious disease affecting fish was described in 1682 and possibly in the 15th century in the Solovetskii islands [27].Remedies against bubonic or pneumonic plague and anthrax included quarantine and in cases of pneumonic or other severe forms of anthrax—the burning of homes, with all their contents, and the burning of infected animals [28]. In the lightest cases of anthrax—boils or carbuncles on the skin that were not lethal--unless cuts on the skin allowed the bacteria to penetrate and attack internal organs--medicinal herbs comprised part or all of the treatment. One treatment involved applying "raisin berries"-- probably dried berries-- to the boil. A stronger treatment involved "pinching" the boil with a heated iron. The wound was then treated with salve, water, and a poultice of herbs [29]. Siberian plague—anthrax--periodically reappeared, as a result of contact with bacterial organisms in the soil that can survive for hundreds of years or as a result of contact with infected deer through skinning their hides or drinking their blood and eating their flesh. Indeed, because the Nenets, reindeer herders of Russian's far north, still indulge in the latter practices and because vaccination of reindeer herds that was mandatory in Soviet times has lapsed, epidemics of anthrax still flare-up [30].

Other epidemics of infectious diseases that periodically recurred in Russia were usually the result of wars, such as the Seven Years War in the second half of the 18th century. A major epidemic of bubonic plague occurred in the early 1770s during Catherine the Great's first war against the Ottoman Empire. High mortality rates, many felling workers in the woolen and silk manufactories of Moscow, coupled with isolation and quarantines, led to major riots in Moscow. The remedies of the day were few. Empress Catherine herself suggested the following herbal remedy: "A capable surgeon should select several hopelessly infected persons. Housed in cool, dry quarters, the sick should be given cold water with vinegar to drink and rubbed with ice at least twice a day," according to John T. Alexander, who has published a tome on the subject [31].

A ray of hope came to Russia and the world with the use of a vaccine against smallpox in the 18th century. Inoculation, long used in India as variolation, which Lady Mary Wortley Montagu observed in Istanbul in 1717, was made safer by Edward Jenner's immunization with cowpox. Empress Catherine the Great eagerly mandated vaccination in Russia, having her son Paul publicly vaccinated—and then herself--as examples [32].

But until the discovery of vaccines for other infectious diseases, the discovery of sulfa drugs and antibiotics in the late 1930s and 1940s, and the re-discovery of phages in the 1930s, Russians' chief weapons against epidemics continued to be isolation, quarantine, liberal use of soap and disinfectants, and for typhus, the Russian steam bath or sauna. Additionally, they applied medicinal plants to strengthen the immune system and to ease the fevers, dehydration, cramps, and diarrhea of cholera, dysentery, and typhoid, the fevers, sweating, and hallucinations of typhus and pneumonia, and the coughing, aches, and other symptoms of influenza and common colds. Many of these plants were rich in protein and vitamins and had bactericide properties. Although these properties were not fully known at the time, the benefits of the botanicals were visible from empirical evidence.

Typhus felled many in Napoleon's Grand Armée as soldiers straggled out of Russia in the fall of 1812 [33]. A cholera epidemic erupted in Russia in 1831-1832. Unfortunately, John Snow's discovery that cholera was spread by polluted water came two decades later, in 1854. Nevertheless, herbal remedies prevented the use of harsh treatments which worsened the impact of cholera, dysentery, and other diarrheal diseases.

Vilma Gudienė, Lithuanian pharmacist and historian of pharmacy noted that Russian court physicians eschewed the harsh bleeding in vogue in Western Europe and the United States in the early 19th century when treating their royal patients [34]. Roderick McGrew, historian of cholera epidemics in Russia, notes that Russian physicians were also reluctant to use bleeding for the treatment of ordinary Russians suffering from cholera in 1831 and 1832. He credits Russian physicians for collecting statistics on the demographics of cholera victims, for theorizing that cholera was caused by a microscopic agent that infiltrated the body, and for realizing that bleeding worsened the condition of the sick [35]. According to McGrew the most famous cure for the symptoms of cholera in the early 1830s was the herbal remedy of Dr. Leo of Warsaw (much of Poland being under Russian control at that time). Dr. Leo's remedy ordained that the cholera patient be given a drink that combined three grains of bismuth, with sugar and Melissa every two to three hours to soothe the stomach. "To counteract muscular cramps, a special liniment was made up from one ounce of liquid *ammoniae causticae* and six ounces of spirits of angelica. The compound was to be applied hot. The combined bismuth and liniment treatment was to be continued until the secretion of urine together with natural body heat returned." [36] McGrew also praises Russian physicians for emphasizing that "the revival of vital energies"--*i.e.* the immune system--of the cholera patient was important. To this end, the patient was given plant items such as opium, ether, salts and spirits of hartshorn, valerian, snakeroot, angelica, arnica–along with camphor, musk, phosphorous and other items [37].

Botanicals in the Imperial Period: 18th and 19th Centuries to 1917

Centralized Control over the Pharmaceutical Sector and Botanicals

The practice of pharmacy in Russia remained highly regulated by the Central Government from the beginning of the Imperial period in the 18th century down to the end of the empire in 1917. Concomitantly, the cultivation of plants, collection of wild plants, and research into plants continued to be important in Russian medicine. Exports of plants from the Russian Empire also was lucrative, as the Russian government had a monopoly on key plant items.

In the first quarter of the 18th century, during the reign of Peter the Great, the Medical Chancellery in the Ministry of Internal Affairs replaced the *Aptekarskii Prikaz* or Pharmacy Department of the Muscovite Period. Situated in Peter's new capital of St. Petersburg, the Medical Chancellery included a Pharmacy Department although all the directors staffing it were physicians, save for one pharmacist—an administration which chaffed pharmacists through until the end of the Empire.

In 1716, Peter also established a medical garden on Apothecary Island in St. Petersburg. The garden was laid out according to the "Vertograd," a Lithuanian translation in 1534 of a German manual which had first appeared in Lübeck in 1492. This manual detailed plants native to Russia and their applications although the names of the plants were usually given in Latin, Greek, and German, sometimes in Arabic, rarely in Polish, and rarely in Russian [38].

The Russian Government also established a monopoly on important plants and plant products. From the 17th through the early 19th century a chief botanical export was rhubarb. "Russian" rhubarb gained worldwide fame as a high-quality purgative. Special warehouses culled the plants and exported only the best. The site in eastern Siberia where the rhubarb originated was a closely guarded state secret [39].

Government-regulated health care and dispensing also expanded in Russia. In 1775, following the bubonic plague and her first war against the Ottoman Empire, Empress Catherine the Great implemented the "Guberniia Reform." This reform organized the European part of the Empire into approximately 50 provinces, each divided into 10 districts, based on population and governed by an appointed Governor. Boards of Welfare were established in each province to handle epidemic diseases and establish hospitals, schools, insane asylums, and old age homes. The Boards hired medical experts. Networks of pharmacies—mostly privately owned but closely scrutinized by the Medical Chancellery--fanned out across the Empire even in the cities of Siberia [40]. Medical schools were established in Russia in the 18th and 19th centuries, the first being the Military Medical Academy in St. Petersburg. By the late 19th century eleven universities operated in the Russian Empire, some in Siberian cities.

Scientific Research of the 18th and early 19th Centuries on Botanicals Used Against Infectious Diseases, Including Plants Used in Popular Medicine (Narodnaia meditsina) by Russians and non-Russian Inhabitants of the Russian Empire

Russian physicians and pharmacologists did important research on plants in the 18th and 19th centuries. Hundreds of articles and books describing research on the properties and application of botanicals not only in the entire Russian Empire but in specific provinces are listed in the *Bibliography on Medicinal Plants* published by the Academy of Sciences of the Soviet Union in 1957. One of the most interesting aspects of this research is that, in the 18th and 19th centuries, academics who did research on plants, included not only studies done in their laboratories but the use of plants by "simple people." This would remain the case in the Soviet period of the 20th century, when for instance, as we will see later in this chapter, during World War II Soviet pharmacologists studied plants used in popular medicine. At this point, amongst the plethora of books and articles that appeared during the 18th and 19th centuries on the use of various plants for medicinal purposes, we will only mention some of the most important publications specifically dealing with infectious diseases.

In the second half of the 18th century, Tobias E. Lovits, who immigrated to Russia from Gottigen and apprenticed at the Court Pharmacy in St. Petersburg, was known for his research on charcoal. He devised a quick method of purifying tartaric acid with charcoal. Some of his findings were used to make potable water for the Russian army and navy [41].

One of the most important 18th-century Russian specialists on medicinal botanicals was A. T. Bolotov, editor of the journal *Ekonomicheskii magazin* (Economic store) from 1780-1789. He wrote and published hundreds of articles on the use of plants for medical problems and diseases—some infectious. He admitted that he could not ascertain the effectiveness of the measures published in the journal but asked his readers to expound on and verify these measures [42]. Indeed the efficacy of many of the remedies discussed by Bolotov and his contemporaries has been proven not only by continued usage of the plants but by examination of the properties of these botanicals in modern laboratories. For example, in 1780, in an article on the use of botanicals to counter diarrhea, Bolotov advocated powders made from xvoshch (*Equisètum*) and the roots of zmeevik (*Rhizoma Bistortae*, family *Polygonaceae*). Among other components, xvoshch contains the alkaloids nicotine, flavonoids, five glucosides of liuteolin, small percentages of vitamin C and carotene--harmful to those with lung cancer but otherwise beneficial, aconite acid and other acids, and about 16 percent protein, and fatty oils. Zmeevik roots contain up to 25 percent tannic acid and up to 26 percent starch. The ingredients in zmeevik, thus, would stop diarrhea. Those in xvoshch would supply electrolytes and nutrition to the patient. The roots of zmeevik also were valued for their hemostatic and anti-inflammatory properties [43]. In 1783, to combat chest colds and coughs, Bolotov recommended the juice of an onion, camphor, and syrup of Moscow vodka, wine made from berries and sugar [44]. To counter inflammation from mosquitoes—annoying at that time and later discovered to be vectors of many infectious diseases--Bolotov suggested washing the skin with artemisia or with tmin (*Carum carvi* L.) or caraway seeds, boiled in vinegar wine. An article published in 2013 in *Research in Pharmaceutical Sciences* supports Bolotov, stating: "Vapors from caraway seeds have been effective in relieving pain and inflammation in patients suffering from lumbar pains and rheumatism." The article also notes additional medicinal uses: "Caraway has also been used in bronchopulmonary disorders as cough remedy and demulcent." Additionally, there are numerous studies about" *Carum carvi* L. for treating "gastrointestinal disorders." [45]

In 1792 the scholarly researcher, I. I. Lepekhin, provided data on 25 plants used in popular medicine against fevers and venereal diseases [46]. Unfortunately, no details are available.

A. P. Neliubin, one of the most noteworthy pharmacists of the early 19th century, came from the far northern provincial city of Viatka but made his mark in St. Petersburg, the capital of the Russian Empire. He received the degree of Provisor or full-fledged pharmacist in 1805. He served as a city obstetrician and helped formulate the *Aptekarskaia taksa*—a schedule of prices for which pharmaceuticals were to be dispensed, but also managed to do useful pharmaceutical research. Having been appointed to the Medical Council in the Ministry of Internal Affairs, the government sent him to the Caucasus to study mineral waters. As a member of the St. Petersburg Pharmaceutical Society, founded in 1818, Neliubin invented a method of deriving salts of quinine and created an apparatus for making ether and analyzing arsenic. One of his textbooks that described the nomenclature and description of new medicinal substances went through five editions. Another text, published in 1831, discussed foreign proprietary medicines imported from abroad and domestic proprietary medicines—which were few—the Russian government prohibiting most. For example, Neliubin dismissed one antipyretic, a universal remedy of the time containing *macilaginem gummi Tragacanthae* and sugar, declaring that nothing could be expected from its use [47].

A contemporary of Neliubin, A. M. Butlerov discovered two alkaloids. He derived "urotropine" in 1859 and studying the structure of quinine, discovered "khinoline." He also synthesized saccharin from formaldehyde. So much research was done on quinine in Russia because, as noted, malaria was endemic and sometimes epidemic through the 20th century up to the northern regions of Russia as well as in the south and the Caucasus [48].

In 1832, a book on popular medicine in Ukraine was translated from French into Russian. In the same year, one A. Levshin published a book "about diseases and treatment with herbs" amongst the Turkic Kirgiz-Kazakh hordes of the Siberian steppes, the latter nomadic peoples having come under Russian control in the second half of the 18th century [49].

In 1835, amongst numerous studies on plants, an article in the journal *Drug zdraviia* (Friend of Health) discussed the application of the roots of *Sonnoi odura* in three cases of scarlet fever. I have not been able to locate information on this plant. Articles by E. Smel'skii in that same journal discussed the use of *Artemisia vulgaris* in cases of convulsions among children lasting more than three days and the use of cabbage in cases of vomiting. Regarding the serious convulsions, modern research has shown that in addition to vermifuge properties, *Artemisia* contains betaine, choline, tannins, and other compounds. Betaine and Choline are essential to health. Betaine helps with digestion by helping the body break down foods. It helps increase stomach acid, improves liver function and helps against anemia. Choline is important for liver function and cell structure. It also has anti-inflammatory properties [50].

Another article published in 1835 reviewed the use of Extract *Pulsatillae* for coughs among children. *Pulsatilla* is a homeopathic product sold on the internet at the present time. An 1836 article in *Drug zdraviia* by one Shianna discussed the use of black pepper for fever and bloody diarrhea. Articles in this journal regarding the use of botanicals to treat diarrhea continued to be prominent from 1838 to 1841. Diarrhea was a major killer of children in Russia in the 19th century and debilitated adults suffering from dysentery and cholera. In 1838, an article by Arnold recommended syrup of cheremukhi (*Prunus padus or Bird Cherry*) for diarrhea in children as well as an infusion of black cherries. In 1840 an article by one Ivanov again advocated the roots of *Prunus padus* for diarrhea as did an article in 1841 by one Budberg. A modern 21-page article published in 2020 in *Nutrients*, entitled "Phytopharmacological Possibilities of Bird Cherry *Prunus padus L.* and *Prunus serotine L.* Species and their Bioactive Phytochemicals" by Aleksandra Telichowska, Joanna Kobus-Cisowska and Piotr Szulc, confirms the correctness of the usage of this plant against diarrhea in Russia in the 1840s. The modern researchers note that wild cherry contains tannins. These stop diarrhea. Wild cherry also contains carbohydrates, glucose, fructose, and sorbitol. The seeds contain magnesium and have high protein content. *Prunus padus L.* contains Tocopherols and Vitamin C—thus replenishing nutrients lost in bouts of diarrhea. "P. padus," the article continues, "is a source of flavonols…used as a food ingredient or…for production of supplements," Further, the authors note that Bird Cherry has antioxidant properties. and antimicrobial activity [51].

A number of articles in Russian journals appearing between 1853 and 1854 dealt with cholera and fever—perhaps due to the outbreak of the Crimean War in 1853 that pitted Russia against the Ottoman Empire, Britain, France, and Piedmont, Italy. The roots of sumbul or *Ferula moschata* were recommended by an anonymous author in 1853 in the *Proceedings of the Military Economic Society*. Wikipedia gives the plant, native to Turkestan and Central Asia, short shrift, stating it has a bitter taste and is mainly used for food preservation and also for perfumes. In contrast, an article by Poonam Mahendra and Shadra Bisht in *Pharmacognosy Review*, 2012, highly praises *Ferula asafoetida*, a traditional medicinal botanical in India, Afghanistan, China, and other countries near Russia. Mahendra and Bisht relate that *Ferula asafoetida* is used orally for hysteria and whooping cough. The decoction of the plant is applied as a vermifuge in China. In Saudi Arabia, *Ferula* is used to treat whooping cough, asthma, and bronchitis. In Egypt "Hot water extract of the dried root is taken orally as an antispasmodic, a diuretic, a vermifuge and an analgesic" and is "claimed to be a powerful antispasmodic in the United States." [52] In 1853, S. Lavrent'ev advocated *Acorus calamus* against fevers. According to Wikipedia, although this plant has been used from the time of the ancient Egyptians, in Europe, and by some American Indians, "there is no clinical evidence for its safety or efficacy—and ingested calamus may be toxic—leading to its commercial ban in the United States." [53] Apparently, many users in 19th century Russia thought differently.

In 1854 Russian researcher V. Boborykin advocated "Shipovnik—*Rosa Rogusa*—as a remedy for fevers." The medicinal properties of this plant, touted in early Russian manuscripts, were confirmed in the 1970s and 1980s, as noted earlier in the present chapter. More recent science continues to proclaim the benefits of *Rosa rogusa* in general and for countering the symptoms of infectious diseases. A current internet article on Ramanas Rose or *Rosa rogusa* states: "The leaves are used in the treatment of fevers. The flowers act on the spleen and liver, promoting blood circulation….The root is used in the treatment of coughs. The fruit of many members of this genus (Rosaceae) is a very rich source of vitamins and minerals, especially in vitamins A, C and E, flavonoids and other bio-active compounds. It also is a fairly good source of essential fatty acids." Further, the modern article states, the plant is "being investigated for halting the growth of cancers." [54] In 1854 two articles in the Russian journal *Proceedings of the Military Economic Society* advocated *Inula Helenium* against chestotka—or "itch" and *Helianthus tuberosus* against whooping cough. Modern science does not specifically recommend *Helianthus tuberosus* (Jerusalem artichoke) against whooping cough but notes that the plant "is used as a digestif and as a remedy for diarrhea or abdominal pain." [55] An extract of another herb mentioned in early Russian manuscripts, boligolova (*Conium*), also was recommended in 1854 in an article in the Russian journal of the Free Economy Society, to treat whooping cough. Modern science is ambivalent about this remedy. The website of CAB International admits that *Conium maculatum* "was said to relieve coughing from bronchitis, whooping cough and asthma" (Botanical com, 2015) but warns that this was an early 20th-century remedy and at present, it is dismissed because of dangerous properties [56].

To conclude, this survey of Russian research in the 18th and early 19th centuries on botanicals for use against infectious diseases mainly has stood the test of time and been shown to be sensible.

Scientific Research on Botanicals in the Second Half of the 19th Century and Early 20th Century

Russian research on botanicals continued in the latter 19th century, becoming even more scientifically grounded. Georg Dragendorff was one of the most important pharmacists conducting plant research during this period. He was born in 1836 in Rostok, apprenticed in a pharmacy, and after taking the requisite examinations, became a fully-qualified pharmacist or Provisor in 1858. He studied two years at Heidelburg University, worked in a chemical laboratory at Rostok University, and received a Doctor of Philosophy degree from that university in 1861. Dragendorff briefly managed the laboratory of the St. Petersburg Pharmacy Society. In 1864 he was awarded a Magistr of Pharmacy degree from Dorpat University in Estland (present-day Estonia, but at that time a province of the Russian Empire), and was appointed director of the Pharmacy Institute at Dorpat University. He remained at that university as a professor until 1894. His research and that of his students in the 1860s and 1870 were on plant alkaloids. He and his students analyzed quinine, ptomaine, salicylic acid, and ether oil. According to one historian of pharmacy, Dragendorff contributed "importantly to plant chemistry by developing a systematic process of plant analysis, based largely on solvent extraction procedures." [57]

There were other Russian plant researchers of equal ability in the late 19th century. Professor V. A. Tikhomirov, in the department of pharmacy and pharmacognosy at the University of Moscow, did research on the acclimation of foreign herbs and tea to Russia. A. V. Pel', who received a Magistr of Pharmacy Degree from the Military Medical Academy in St. Petersburg in 1873, investigated atropine and other alkaloids, rational methods of preparing galenical mixtures, and aseptic medical procedures. Pel' published 132 scientific studies. He was the first to extract spermine in pure form. A. A. Voznesenskii and N. N. Zinin both of whom died in 1880, isolated the alkaloid theobromine and researched the chemical structure of quinine. In 1889, Magistr of Pharmacy E. A. Shatskii published *Studies on Vegetable Alkaloids, Glucosides, and Ptomaines*. In 1896, Professor E. A. Leman of Tomsk University in western Siberia isolated a glucoside which he called "periplotsin" from the root of *Periploca graeca L.* a substance that had a beneficial effect on heart disease [58].

Dmitrii Ivanovskii, credited with the discovery of viruses, was a botanist whose research began in 1887 on microscopic infectious agents attacking tobacco plants in Ukraine, Bessarabia and then in Crimea [59]. Ivanovsky's mentor was botanist Andrei Famitsyn, who studied under fungal expert Lev S. Tsenkovsky at the University of St. Petersburg. According to a Wikipedia article on him, in 1890 he "founded and headed the Laboratory of Plant Anatomy and Physiology of the [Russian] Academy of Sciences." He published texts on photosynthesis and plant metabolism, "was the first to separate green algae cells from lichen," and to use artificial light for plant growing" [60].

Women pharmacists also contributed to preventing and treating infectious diseases. Although women had been allowed to own pharmacies and wives of pharmacists had assisted in managing pharmacies, women were officially permitted to practice as pharmacists in women's medical facilities only in 1871. In 1888, they were formally allowed to become Assistant Pharmacists—with right of general practice, which required passing government examinations—and also to become Provizors, a title which entailed two years of university study. Several women eagerly entered the field. One of the most famous is Antonina Lesnevskaia, of Polish descent, who established the All Women's Pharmacy on the Nevskii prospect, the main thoroughfare in St. Petersburg in 1901 and in 1903 founded a pharmacy school for women that graduated some 300 by 1913. Ol'ga Evgeniia Gabrilovich wrote her thesis for the title Magistr of Pharmacy in 1906 on her study of the causes of "intoxicating bread" a debilitating disease that felled many individuals who ate rye bread—a staple of the lower classes--in many provinces of Russia. Hired on by zemstvos, her careful and laborious research showed that the problem was a fungus *Fusarium roseum link*, which contained a glucoside that absorbed the protein in rye kernels, thus depriving them of nutrition. In the course of her work Gabrilovich noted the coexistence of mold and bacteria on her Petri dishes, but, unfortunately, did not follow up on what became known as penicillin in the 1920s [61].

Plant-Based Pharmaceuticals *versus* Chemically Synthesized Pharmaceuticals in the Treatment of Infectious Diseases in Late Imperial Russia—1880s to 1917

In the last two decades of the 19th century, the discovery of the etiology of many diseases was paralleled by the production of chemically synthesized medicines—the so-called "magic bullets" produced by Western European pharmaceutical firms to treat infectious diseases. Russian researchers produced vaccines in the early 20th century, but before World War I, Russian pharmaceutical companies in Russia did not produce the "magic bullets." For this reason, Soviet pharmacologists denigrated the Imperial Russian pharmaceutical industry as backward. They claimed that in the last two decades of the 19th century and the first decade of the 20th century—before the advent of Soviet Power in 1917--Russia imported almost all factory-produced medicines from foreign countries—particularly from German and Swiss firms—Merck, Schering, Bayer, Hoffman-La Roche--and from some American firms. This characterization of the Russian pharmaceutical sector is inaccurate. Nevertheless, it has been repeated in countless histories.

It is accurate to admit that before World War I Russia imported the new chemically synthesized pharmaceuticals—the so-called magic bullets like aspirin, phenacetin, the anti-venereal Salvarsan, antipyrine, and Novocain—from Swiss and German pharmaceutical firms. Also imported were five plant-based products--quinine, cocaine, iodine, opiates, and the hemostatic *Hydrastis canadensis*—for reasons given below [62]. However, Russia—as did the United States at the time—imported these items for logical reasons as well as because of pre-existing conditions. Further, the products of the Russian pharmaceutical industry—particularly soap and disinfectants—were important for combatting infectious diseases of the time and improving the health of the population.

At the outset of this rebuttal, it should be emphasized that late Imperial Russia did not lack chemists, a chemical industry, laboratories, and pharmaceutical factories. Chemistry had become a specialized study in Russia from the 18th century. Russians, like the polymath Mikhail Lomonosov and his successors, soon excelled in that field—as did Pafnuty Chebyshev at the University of St. Petersburg and Nikolai Lobachevsky at the University of Kazan in the fields of mathematics. In 1841, Russian chemist Nicholai Zinin produced a compound from nitrobenzene—aniline—that became the base for synthetic dyes and for synthetic drugs. Large- scale production of pharmaceuticals began in Russian Poland in the first half of the 19th century. In Russia proper, A. A. Andreev established a steam-powered laboratory for pharmaceutical preparations in Moscow in 1862 [63]. Russian chemical and pharmaceutical factories increased exponentially in the 1870s, 1880s, and 1890s. By 1913, approximately 300 chemical factories—many small but some very large-- operated in the Russian Empire. Before World War I, Russian factories and workshops produced salicylic acid, the base for aspirin, benzol, phenol, and almost all the aniline used in the Empire. Approximately 100 pharmaceutical factories—some very large--operated in the Russian Empire, supplying disinfectants, soap, cough syrups, and the like to combat and treat the symptoms of infectious diseases. Separate institutes supplied vaccines against typhus, typhoid, dysentery, and other infectious diseases [64]. Pharmacies—the organization of which shall be discussed shortly—compounded many medicines in house. However, they also procured medicines from Russian pharmaceutical companies as well as from foreign pharmaceutical firms. Some zemstvo pharmacies (defined shortly) acquired half or more of the medicines they dispensed from Russian firms. Put another way, Russian firms produced 7 million (gold backed) rubles' worth of pharmaceutical products in comparison with 3 million rubles' worth of medicines that were imported [65].

Nevertheless, Russian-made pharmaceuticals consisted of plant-based, hormonal, and mineral products, salves that were by-products of Russia's booming oil industry, cleaning agents, substances for preserving foods, dried foods that were bases for soups, fruit, mineral-water and milk drinks like those produced by Nestlé, cough syrups, bandages, surgical and medical apparatus, shampoos and perfumes—in addition to the toilet and laundry soaps and detergents cited above. Many of these products were of high quality, received gold medals at foreign exhibitions, and were featured in glossy colored advertisements [66]. Further, rural dwellers—who comprised 80 percent of the population—relied heavily on plant remedies that they concocted themselves.

Russia imported the chemically synthesized "magic bullets" from foreign firms because of geographical conditions and for economic and legal considerations.

Firstly, the Russian Empire abounded in medicinal plants. Russia did need to import quinine against malaria, as has been mentioned above. She also needed to import cocaine. Although opium poppies grew in Russia and although Russia had ample coasts for iodine--important as an antidote to goiter and as a disinfectant against infectious diseases like typhus, typhoid, dysentery, cholera, and so on—the active ingredients in Russian poppies and Russian seaweed did not satisfy the Russian pharmacopoeia. Therefore, before the First World War, opium or opiates were imported from Persia and the Ottoman Empire; iodine, produced from Chilean seaweed, was imported from Germany. V. K. Ferrein, the owner of one of the largest pharmaceutical factories in Russia and the largest pharmacy in the world, tried to grow *Hydrastis canadensus*—a hemostatic—on his plantation outside Moscow but was forced to import this plant from the United States [67].

Otherwise, medicinal plants were cultivated and collected on a wide scale in Siberia as well as European Russia in the 19th and early 20th centuries by peasants as well as on estates. The business was lucrative. In the 1840s and 1850s, the marketing of caraway seed oil, derived from *Virtuca virosa*, and mustard oil was big business in Ukraine [68]. In the second half of the 19th century one of the main centers of plant cultivation was in Voronezh province; cultivation of anise, coriander and chernushka (*Nigella arvensis L.*), rich in Vitamin C, occupied up to 3,000 *dessiatinas* (about the same amount of hectares or 8,000 acres) in one district alone. In Tula province, the cultivation of sage and chamomile occupied 100 *dessiatinas*. In Poltava Province cultivation of mint occupied up to 1,000 dessiatinas in two districts. In Podolia Province cultivation of fennel or *Foeniculum officinale* occupied up to 200 dessiatinas. In the lower Volga region cultivation of mustard occupied up to 2,000 dessiatinas. *Artemisia cina* grew only near Chimkent, in Russian Turkestan [69].

Plants were not only widely used in popular medicine in the 19th and early 20th centuries but were major exports, even during World War I. For example, chief Russian exports to the United States included licorice root, sporyn'e (*Secale cornutum*)—a fungus on roses, and lycopodium (*Sporae likopodii*) or club moss. From the 1880s, Russia also had a monopoly on Santonin, the round-worm expellant produced from *Artemisia cina*, that was vital to the American hog industry. In 1913, Russia exported 1,000 tons of medicinal plants valued at 436,000 gold rubles [70].

A second reason for widespread, longstanding use of medicinal plants was the fact that the vast majority of the Russian populace lived in the countryside whereas the vast majority of pharmacies and medical clinics were located in urban areas. In contrast to Britain and the United States, the Russian government strictly controlled the pharmaceutical sector. A Medical Board in the Ministry of Internal Affairs certified pharmacists as well as physicians and closely supervised the pharmaceutical sector. There were two kinds of pharmacies. "Normal" pharmacies were fully stocked and managed by a fully qualified pharmacist, a *Provizor,* who had apprenticed in a pharmacy, taken university courses, and passed government certification examinations. Pharmacists in normal pharmacies compounded as well as sold factory-prepared medicines. Normal pharmacies were open around the clock. The prices for medicines dispensed were regulated by the government through the so-called *Aptekarskaia taksa* although pharmacies often gave out medicine free to the poor. The government scrutinized the architecture of pharmacies, the rooms in which dried medicines and other products were stored, preparation rooms, and so on and fined pharmacies that did not meet the test. Thus, the quality of Russian dispensing was good. Unfortunately, it was not easy to establish a normal pharmacy, even if one had ample money to do so. To prevent undue competition, the Russian government established population norms, distance from other pharmacies, and permission from owners of already existing pharmacies as criteria for the establishment of a new pharmacy. In rural areas, the pharmacies were partially stocked and managed by a partially trained pharmacist or even a non-pharmacist because fully trained pharmacists and doctors did not want to live in the countryside [71].

Zemstvos were established in 34 internal provinces in 1864 in order to bring more pharmacies to rural areas. The zemstvos replaced the Boards of Health established in the 18th century by Catherine the Great in these 34 provinces. Like the Boards of Health, they were mandated to care for local health, educational and infrastructure needs. Zemstvos collected taxes from property owners to do so. As a result, local property owners had more representation in the zemstvos than had been the case in the Boards of Health. Property owners were grouped into three categories to elect representatives to the district zemstvo. The first group included owners of real property and businesses--a category that included mainly nobles but also non-nobles—even peasants. The second category included townspeople with property. The third category included peasants, who were holders of communal property. The district zemstvo then elected representatives to the provincial zemstvo. Zemstvo pharmacies were established in the capital city of the province and in each of the approximately 10 districts that comprised the province. By the early 20th century there were only about 200 zemstvos pharmacies. They competed with private pharmacies, however, by often dispensing medicines at prices lower than those set in the *Aptekarskaia taksa*—or entirely free—not only to zemstvo taxpayers but to all in the vicinity. In other words, the zemstvo pharmacies practiced socialized pharmacy—whereas the private pharmacies had to make a profit as well as serve the public need [72].

In the early 20th century a network of approximately 4,800 pharmacies operated in Russia. However, some 2,845 of these pharmacies were located in cities—even in Siberian cities—whereas only 1,825 lesser stocked pharmacies served the countryside where 80 percent of the population lived [73]. The zemstvo pharmacies were supposed to solve this problem but most of the 200 zemstvo pharmacies were mainly in cities [74]. The shortage of pharmacies, even in the cities, resulted in so-called "drugstores"—that could sell factory-made pharmaceuticals and sundries but not compound medicines. By 1910 they were twice as numerous as pharmacies [75].

Thus, in the countryside, peasants self-medicated with time-honored remedies. Household staples included citric acid and grape juice to treat bronchial catarrh and bronchitis as well as chronic urinary disorders. Vinegar acid was used against fever and scarlatina as well as to help the auto-immune problem eczema. *Fructus*

Foeniculi was used as an expectorant in colds and flu as well as for digestive problems in newborns, in small doses to increase breast milk and in larger doses for hemorrhaging from the womb and to prevent miscarriage. *Herba origani* "grown all over Russia," was used for toothache; camphor was dispensed for cases of typhus and cholera as well as for heart disease. The oil and acid of valerian root, grown all over Russia, was used to treat the symptoms of typhus and to kill worms--as well as to calm nervous diseases. Artemisia root, also common in Russia, was used in contractions of the womb (and from the 1880s to make the round-worm expellant Santonin). Siberian castor also was used to treat problems of the womb. Tannin was used to treat digestive problems, kidney problems and diarrhea. The latter could arise from infectious diseases as well as spoiled food [76].

Third, patents and financial considerations influenced Russia's import of foreign chemically synthesized medicines. Foreign firms held the patents for the new "magic bullets," such as aspirin and Salvarsan, to combat syphilis. Additionally, import tariffs between Russia and Germany were low after 1905. Thus, despite Russia having a pharmaceutical industry that produced about half the factory-made pharmaceuticals—many of high quality--dispensed in the empire, it was more economical for Russia to import the foreign chemically synthesized medicines than to reverse engineer and produce analogs of them domestically. Even some of the 200 zemstvo pharmacies that practiced socialized dispensing ordered half or all their medicines from Russian firms [77].

Finally, the glacial slowness at which the Russian government assayed and approved new medicines also held back the Russian pharmaceutical industry. Before his untimely assassination in 1911, Peter Arkad'evich Stolypin, Minister of Internal Affairs, tried to make the Russian pharmaceutical industry more competitive. He proposed producing Russian versions of foreign preparations as long as the domestic items were labeled "Made in Russia." This outraged German, Swiss, and French pharmaceutical companies, and the proposal went nowhere [78].

World War I: Medicines for Infectious Diseases

During the First World War, though, cut off from German and Swiss imports, Russian pharmacists and pharmacologists did reverse-engineer some of the key chemically-synthesized medicines-- aspirin, Salvarsan, Novocain, phenacetin and others—to quell the symptoms of head colds, influenza, Syphilis, and other infectious diseases. These Russian-made "magic bullets" were used by the imperial family, as the *signatury* or labels on their medicine bottles attest--and also dispensed to the general population [79].

In addition, cultivation and collection of medicinal plants not only continued but became a crusade. For example, ordinary citizens, including schoolchildren, were instructed to collect medicinal botanicals. The botanical product, Peruvian Balsam, made from the tree *Myroxylon balsamum var. pereirae* found in El Salvador, was imported. But, cut off from foreign sources of opium and iodine, as the Ottoman Empire and Germany were now Russia's enemies, domestic opium poppies and Black Sea seaweed were used during the war. The great danger to the Russian soldiers during the First World War--15 million men being mobilized--were infectious diseases. Typhoid and cholera broke out the first year of the war; in succeeding years dysentery, croupous inflammation of the lungs, malaria, scabies, and impetigo sickened and killed troops. Many remedies were produced from minerals or petroleum products--coal-tar salves, sulfur salves, hydrogen peroxide, hydrochloric acid, kerosene, and benzine. Iodine, produced from niter or saltpeter and seaweed, was a crucial item at the front and the production of Russian iodine grew exponentially. Tincture of iodine was used as a topical disinfectant and also to disinfect water. Forty-five to 50 percent of wounds suffered by Russian soldiers were to soft tissue and in 1915 one M. V. Rostovtsev developed a special apparatus to treat these wounds with iodine steam which he recommended in place of infusions of iodine. Previously imported from Germany, which produced iodine from Chilean sources, iodine production in Russia rose to 2,000 puds (72,000 pounds) or 36 tons by mid-1916. The measures to strengthen Russia's pharmaceutical industry brought results. Two and ½ million troops perished but unusual mortality was low amongst civilians [80].

THE SOVIET PERIOD

The Civil War and Infectious Disease Epidemics in Belarus, 1922-1923

During the Civil War of 1917-1921, on the other hand, an estimated 11 and ½ million people perished—most civilians—in great part due to infectious diseases. Typhus was the big killer, but typhoid, cholera, recurring fever, dysentery, and malaria were scourges as well [81]. Epidemics of these same infectious diseases continued to rack Belarus during 1922-23 due to huge numbers of refugees and transients. The latter included those returning to the nascent Soviet Union and those trying to leave. The former referred to Soviet citizens fleeing from famine in the Volga River region, Ukraine, and North Caucasus. The American Relief Association (ARA) under Herbert Hoover gave enormous assistance to Belarus [82] as well as to the famine-stricken provinces [83]. In 1925, the Soviet Union still registered a very high incidence of these infectious diseases compared with Germany and other Western European countries [84].

Return to *narodnaia meditsina* and self-medication with medicinal plants became the norm for survival during the civil war and continued in the 1920s and 1930s due to severe shortages of medicines, pharmacies, and pharmacists. The reasons for the shortages have been discussed in my book, *The Soviet Pharmaceutical Business during the First Two Decades, 1917-1937*. Bern, New York: Peter Lang, 2006, so only a short summary will be given in the chapter.

Important pharmaceutical factories had been located in Poland and Latvia; their independence, thus, eliminated two sources of medicines to Bolshevik Russia, Vicious battles between antagonists—the Red Army, armies of various anti-Bolshevik, Socialist groups, White armies comprised of former tsarist soldiers and Cossacks, armies of warlords—that rent European Russia, Ukraine, Belarus, the North Caucasus, and Siberia during the civil war destroyed agricultural land as well as infrastructure. The Peace of Riga that followed the Polish--Belarusian—Russian War of 1919-1920, deprived Bolshevik Russia and Bolshevized Belarus of small-scale chemical, pharmaceutical, footwear, and clothing workshops. However, the policies of "War Communism," that the Bolsheviks implemented after their takeover of the government in October 1917, were more detrimental to pharmacies, pharmaceutical factories, and the cultivation and sale of medicinal botanicals than military operations. Private production and marketing became a crime. The Bolsheviks' seized peasant produce for the Red Army, causing decline of production of food and medicinal botanicals on the part of peasants and limited availability for the general populace. Bolshevik policies crippled the pharmaceutical industry which had grown more self-sufficient by the end of the First World War. Major pharmaceutical factories were nationalized; lesser ones were sequestered by local workers. The factories were mismanaged, and some had no management whatsoever, resulting in neglect and destruction of machinery and stores of materials—disinfectants, soap, cough syrups, and medicines. Pharmacies and "drug-stores" also were sequestered [85]. Trained pharmacists were barred from owning their pharmacies. The number of pharmacies shrank. For example, the number of pharmacies in the entire Belarusian SSR in 1922 was the same as that in Minsk city and province alone during World War I. Caches of medicines in private and public warehouses disappeared [86].

The "New Economic Policy" of the 1920s and the Five-Year Plans, 1928 - 1930s

The Soviet pharmaceutical industry made a comeback during the "New Economic Policy" of the 1920s as described in detail in my book, *The Soviet Pharmaceutical Business during Its First Two Decades*, based on materials from Russian archives and information from Soviet pharmacy journals of the period. However, the industry was still dependent upon foreign inputs and foreign machinery and apparatus. Shortages of raw materials and packaging and a lack of qualified workers held the industry back.

The Soviet Union possessed brilliant virologists, bacteriologists, pharmacologists, and other medical and pharmaceutical researchers. Innovative research on phages was done. The Soviet pharmaceutical industry produced medicines and vaccines comparable to other European countries as detailed in my book, *The Soviet Pharmaceutical Business during Its First Two Decades*. Nevertheless, the industry was never able to fully supply the new factory towns and the growing urban population with factory-produced medicines. During the Five-Year-Plan period of the late 1920s and 1930s, an added problem was that government funding was channeled into large-scale infrastructure projects such as dams, canals, and buildup of the steel industry, leaving scant funds on hand for the pharmaceutical sector. Money for these projects came from sales of Soviet art and antique treasures, and from large exports of grain, medicinal botanicals, and chemicals. Collectivization of peasant agricultural land and animals, combined with crop shortages due to poor weather and excessive exports of grain, resulted in famine in Ukraine, the Caucasus and other areas of the Soviet Union in the early 1930s and in Kazakhstan in the mid-1930s. Large exports of medicinal botanicals and chemicals led to shortages of raw materials to produce medicines in the USSR. Constant reorganization, diverting parts of the pharmaceutical industry to other sectors, and demanding more from the industry by the central government caused further problems. The result was that during the late 1920s and 1930s factory-made medicines were not always available. Thus, Soviet citizens continued to rely on self-medication using medicinal plants they grew or collected on a small scale. Medical treatment was negligible or non-existent for citizens who found themselves in Stalin's labor camps. For the general population, pharmacologists investigated simple popular medicine cures from the 19th and early 20th centuries, including the use of easily acquired medicinal botanicals, to offset the shortages of factory-produced medicines and disinfectants [87].

A Return to Popular Medicine and Botanicals during the Five-Year Plans

During the First Five-Year Plan shortages of iodine, an important disinfectant and antidote for goiter led pharmacologists to investigate the home-made remedy "Iodtannin". This product diluted a spiritous solution of iodine with tannin or milk. Pharmacologists also recommended sea cabbage, which contained iodine, as a food. In 1929 the Ukrainian commissariat of Health resurrected "Brilliant Green," developed in 1907, as an alternative antiseptic to iodine to counter infectious diseases. Another solution was to use iodine residue, an idea that had arisen during the Great War. Finally, Gosmedtorgprom, the agency that ran the pharmaceutical industry, promoted Bromferron, informing the public that this product could be acquired over the counter "in all pharmacies and *sanmagaziny* (drug stores)" as a replacement for iodine [88].

Scientists conducted expeditions across the Soviet Union to look for new medicinal botanicals, touting, for example, *Anabasis aphylla*, *Leontice ewersmanii*, and *Lupinus luteus*. These plants had been discovered by an expedition to Kazakhstan in 1926 and were fully researched by 1929. Three expeditions took place in 1930 to the Altai and Baikal regions of eastern Siberia, to Tibet, to Issak-kul, and to the Caucasus. In 1930, fifteen plants from Central Asia were studied. Twelve were isolated; two yielded alkaloids. In 1931 and 1932, pharmacologists investigated pustyrnik (*Leonorus cardiac* L.). In 1930 a new Soviet joint-stock company, Lektekhsyr'e, published information about the cultivation of henbane (belena), stramonium or thornapple (durmana) and nettles (krapiva)—old standbys not only from the 19th century but from early Russian herbals--with plans to promote these plants for domestic use and export.

Very importantly, as in the Imperial period, large-scale cultivation of medicinal botanicals resumed. State farms (*sovkhozy*) of 500 hectares in Ukraine, 800 hectares in the North Caucasus, and plantations in Tula and Zhitomir grew medicinal botanicals. In 1931, a *sovkhoz* of 5,000 hectares and another of 2,000 hectares were established in the lower Volga region.

The practical result was that 32 new Soviet products appeared in 1932: Sekkakornin –a standardization of sporyn'e, Frangulen—a standardized product from buckthorn, pyrimidine, antipyrine, Phenacetin, veronal, styrichnine, Hydrokhinon—a substitute for quinine, and vanillin. Other hormones and mineral products were produced. Unfortunately, the production of soap—the first defense against infectious diseases, remained low [89].

Popular Medicine and Botanicals during the Second World War, 1939-1945, for Infectious Diseases

For the Soviet Union, World War II unfolded in two stages. From September 1939 until the Soviet Union was invaded June 22, 1941, the Soviet Union was on the offensive—in Poland, in the so-called Winter War with Finland which ended in March 1940, and the Baltic States, primarily from the summer of 1940. Soviet pharmaceutical factories were producing the antimalarial, Akrikhin, sulfa drugs, and bactericide drugs by this time although production was uneven due to irregular deliveries of raw materials, unhygienic conditions in the factories, worker problems, and so on [90].

During the Great Patriotic War, the war on Soviet territory between June 1941 and 1945, the Soviet pharmaceutical industry as well as the citizenry were in difficult straits. As the German army pushed eastward pharmaceutical factories in harm's way evacuated much of their production and workers to Siberia. This was, of course, time-consuming, and disrupted production. Meanwhile, infectious diseases threatened (*i.e.*--the populace.) [91].

The thirty-five-volume work *Opyt sovetskoi meditsiny v Velikoi Otechestvennoi Voiny, 1941-1945,* published under the general editorship of E. I. Smirnov, Minister of Health, gave few statistics on morbidity and mortality but did provide information on diseases and medical problems, and pharmaceuticals to combat them. Dysentery, typhus, and malaria were most pernicious to the troops between 1941-1943, dysentery affecting two-thirds of the Red Army. Typhus affected 26.24 percent, with pneumonia as a complication. Typhus, typhoid and scarlatina were major problems for civilians. As food and housing deteriorated outbreaks of tularemia occurred [92].

A new vaccine for typhus had been developed in 1942. Soap was in short supply but disinfecting chambers—used in the 1920s—compensated to some extent. Iodine was still important, as were Liuminal, Urotropin, narcotic ether, Pyrimidon, and some other "older" products. Production of basic, chemically synthesized medicines--aspirin, Novocain, caffeine, salicylic acid, glucose and insulin—and the new bactericide and sulfa drugs, Streptotsid and Sulfodin, was poor during the first two years of the war. Output increased in 1943. However, "imports" of crucial medicines and medical apparatus were still needed. These were largely lend-lease items from the United States [93].

Botanicals had been investigated in 1938 and 1939, as in previous decades. For example, researchers concluded that Methyl anabasin was an improvement on anabasin, derived from *Anabasis aphylla,* for use as a respiratory stimulant. This product favorably compared with other plant products—lobeline, caffeine, ephedrine, and pilocarpine. *Bidens tripartitus chereda*, first investigated in 1912, was again investigated to treat tuberculosis of the lymph nodes. Oleander [oleandrin, discovered by a Russian research in the 1850s] and Magnolia were researched for use against cardiac problems, skin diseases, malaria, and for use as a diuretic [94].

During the Great Patriotic War, beleaguered Soviet citizens—whether under enemy attack or evacuated to Kazakhstan and Central Asian Republics—were forced by circumstances to self-medicate with medicinal botanicals that they grew on a small scale or collected in the wild. Additionally, Soviet pharmacologists also investigated and promoted medicinal plants used in popular "*narodnaia*" medicine. This story is told in my book, *Medicines for the Soviet Masses during World War II*. Lanham, New York, Toronto: University Press of America, 2008. Therefore, only the pertinent chapters on *narodnaia meditsina* for infectious diseases will be cited.

Chapter 9 opens with this statement: Traditional remedies became a firm fixture of Soviet mainstream medicine during the Great Patriotic War along with the revival of traditions in other sectors." [95] Soviet citizens made soap at home and formulated other medical recipes. Pharmacologists also continued to investigate popular remedies, many time-honored. The book cites interviews with people who were teenagers or adults during the war.

The first two years of the War—September 1939-June 21, 1941--before Russia was invaded—are covered in Chapter 4. Access to factory-made pharmaceuticals varied. Malaria was a major infectious disease during the war. In 1935 the Akrikhin Factory had been built in Moscow to supply akrikhin, a reverse-engineered analog of the German anti-malaria Atabrine [96]. Other chemically synthesized factory products were Red and White Streptotsid and Sulfidin. During the 1930s the Soviet Union developed an antitoxin against scarlatina from the hearts of children who had died from the disease. However, the sister of Dr. David Genis, now residing in Denver, Colorado, died despite receiving this remedy in an infectious hospital. Thus, when David Genis acquired the disease during the war, his mother refused to let him be treated even in the face of threats from Soviet authorities [97]. Other Soviet citizens interviewed in my book remembered that Red Streptotsid was toxic. Therefore, not only because of shortages but because of problems with factory-prepared therapies, many Soviet citizens "Basically" used extracts made from botanicals and fish oil, and also used cupping and mustard plasters to treat infectious as well as chronic diseases. Those interviewed recalled that cardiac-vascular problems and stomach-intestinal problems were treated with naperstanka (foxglove, digitalis) and landysh (lily-of-the-valley) and romashka (chamomile). When Anna Poletspolskaya, as a twelve-year-old girl developed boils all over her body, she was "lubricated with vinegar greens." One woman in Belarus remembered that for sore throats she was treated with the steam from boiled potatoes. Another drank a decoction of carrots when she contracted viral hepatitis. The grandfather of a colleague in Vitebsk, Belarus, used a remedy for his ulcers—an ailment we now know is caused by bacteria---that combined fresh cucumbers and honey [98].

After the Soviet Union was invaded in June 1941, health care became more precarious. *Life and Death in Besieged Leningrad, 1941-44*, edited by John Barber and Andrei Dzeniskevich (Palgrave-Macmillian, 2005) describes the terrible conditions for people trapped in that city. Some of these people later emigrated to Boulder, Colorado, and told me their story of survival. Some citizens voluntarily remained in Moscow. Some in Ukraine lived in dugouts. Tularemia, along with other infectious diseases of wartime, became a problem for them. Many citizens were evacuated to Kazakhstan and Central Asia. Thus, conditions varied for Soviet civilians. Interviews in my book, *Medicines for the Soviet Masses during World War II* cite disparate examples.

Tamara Khaziev, who lived in Ufa in the Bashkir Republic near the Urals, stated that medical and pharmaceutical care was very meager. Most people in her orbit suffered from colds. There were no thermometers to register fevers. However, "shivering strongly was a signal that [body] temperature was raised." People then were treated with herbs. In the winter, leaves of dushitsa or mint leaves boiled in water were applied. In the summer, fresh leaves of dushitsa were used. The sick person also was given "a decoction of dry raspberries, which we gathered ourselves" in order to make them sweat profusely. Another remedy consisted of inserting dry mustard into the nostrils at night and steaming the feet. When there was a great deal of shivering, indicating a high temperature, the body was rubbed with a vinegar essence—100-150 grams of vinegar into one liter of water. For sore throats, one teaspoon of salt was stirred into a glass of boiled water. Chamomile also was boiled and gargled for sore throats, every two or three hours. Ashes from the stove were poured into a bag and affixed to the throat in another remedy for sore throats. For cough, half of a teaspoon of the juice of aloe leaves—grown in a tub or pot in the window-- was drunk two to three times a day. Vishnevskii salve, a product made of fish oil, which had natural disinfecting properties and was available at the pharmacy, was used to prevent infections from cuts and wounds [99].

Soviet citizens evacuated to Kazakhstan and Central Asia appeared to have more access to factory-prepared medicines than Tamara Nikolaeva. But the evacuees also used home-made medicines and made their own soap. Mariiam Samoilovna Tartakovskaya spent the war in Tashkent, Uzbekistan. Aspirin, green soap, and quinine were available. A heart preparation—Strofantan—was factory prepared. However, people also used valerian, lily-of-the-valley (*landysh*) and *naperstank*a (foxglove). Anna Konetspolskaya, who spent the war in a city in Turkmenia, remembers Sul'fidin and aspirin. People also drank warm milk and steamed their feet in hot water. They lubricated wounds with salt and also applied medicinal mud and various berries. They had no toilet soap—but washed with "dark soap" from a local slaughterhouse. Raisa Kuskina's family made their own soap and were lucky enough to have a bathhouse on the collective farms in Kazakhstan where they lived. They ate well due to their kitchen garden and Raisa was given quinine for malaria. When her mother became ill with diarrhea "she was treated with the juice of wild tern." There were no pharmacists but there was a fel'dsher (a sort of medical aide) nearby. People treated themselves with cherries. Liudmila Ravvina in Uzbekistan had access to medicines because her mother worked in a military hospital. Soap, however, was lacking. As a result, clothes were cleaned with ashes.

Dr. David Genis, evacuated to Kzyl-Orda Kazakhstan, remarked that because soap was "deficit" people used wood ash to wash dirty dishes. Indeed, many others interviewed recalled that soap—a major weapon in the arsenal against infectious diseases--was deficit during the war. Maria Sergeevna Kuznetsova grew up in Siberia. For a cold, when it was difficult to breathe, potatoes were boiled in their skins. While still hot, water was poured over the potatoes and the sick person, covered the head with a thick quilt and breathed in the steam.

Others recounted that a dry cough was treated with milk, boiled with an onion. An infusion of dog-rose berries was a good source of Vitamin C. Astonishingly, to eliminate tapeworm, people drank aircraft fuel [100].

As in the First World War, during the Second World War factory workers, Komsomol youth, and school children were put to work to gather pharmaceuticals. A brochure on "Collecting useful Plants" was published in 1942 to help identify and preserve the plants. In 1942 some 1,000 tons of 108 forms of plants were collected—as compared to only 27 forms in 1941. Despite shortages at home, however, in 1942 the USSR [Union of Soviet Socialist Republics] exported 6,809 pounds of belladonna to the United States at a price of 3, 135 dollars. In 1943, the Soviet Union shipped 10, 521 pounds of belladonna to the United States at a price of 4, 431 dollars. Soviet pharmacologists investigated and promoted many botanical remedies. Sweetbriar was recommended against scurvy because it contained Vitamin C. In the 1930s, a drink made of conifer needles was used to obtain Vitamin C; this remedy was used again during the Second World War. Infusions from sweetbriar and conifer needles were sent to treatment institutions and children's homes. In Tomsk in 1942, Drs. EV and VF Korsun relate on pages 234 to 247 of their History of Phytotherapy in Dermatology (Istoriia fitoterapii v dermatologii, Moscow, 2013) that pharmacologists made a salve from Siberian silver fir, the product "KF" from cranberries to treat ulcerating wounds and burns, and used sterile moss in place of deficit bandages. In 1944, an English-language newspaper praised 8,000 tons of herbs gathered under the aegis of the All-Union Medicinal Trust and in 1945 praised the 100,000 acres of botanicals raised on 10,000 collective farms. *Thermopsis* was discovered in the Tien-Shan mountains and used against respiratory ailments [101]. Some dubious remedies also were promoted [102].

HERBALS AGAINST INFECTIOUS DISEASES IN THE SECOND HALF OF THE 20TH CENTURY AND IN THE POST-SOVIET 21ST CENTURY

Problems in the Pharmaceutical Industry

Soviet Pharmacy sector officials helped India develop a pharmaceutical industry after independence in 1948 [103]. However, at home, these officials grappled with many problems as my article "The Soviet Pharmaceutical Industry and Dispensing, 1945-1953, Europe-Asia Studies, 56, 7, November 2004, 963-991, relates. Soviet pharmacy officials were chagrined that in the Seventh Edition of the Soviet Pharmacopoeia, twice as many articles (20.6 percent) were devoted to "natural products"—mainly botanicals—as in the American Pharmacopoeia, whereas articles dealing with organo-therapy, vitamins, vaccines and serums were considerably fewer in the Soviet Pharmacopoeia than in the American Pharmacopoeia (0.51% and 0.34% *versus* 2% and 3% in the American). Industry output varied considerably from the targets dictated by the Five-Year and Annual Plans. Due to lack of mechanization, labor, and distribution problems some regions of the Soviet Union had too much of some medicines and pharmaceutical products, whereas other regions had too little. Thus, citizens continued to rely on self-treatment with botanicals. Soviet pharmaceutical journals contained many articles on medicinal plants. For random examples, there were articles on the alkaloids of sporyn'e, on plants in the Republic of Georgia, on the alkaloids of *Erythrea Centaurium*, on a popular remedy made from the seeds of *Coronilla varia L.* which had digitalis-like properties and was first discovered in 1895, on lobelia, and on plants of the Baikal region to combat inflammation (and infections) of the skin and membranes [104].

Excellent books on the use of botanicals to prevent infectious diseases and treat their symptoms as well as the treatment of chronic medical problems were available in bookstores in the Soviet Union that I purchased in the 1970s and 1980s. One is the Handbook of G. N. Kotukov, Kul'tiruemye i dikorastushchie lekarstvennye rasteniia (Cultivated and Wild Medicinal Plants) published in Kiev by "Naukova dumka" in 1975. The second is A. D. Turova, E. N. Sapozhnikova, Lekarstvennye rasteniia SSSR i ikh primenenie (Medicinal Plants of the USSR and Their Application) published in Moscow by Meditsina, 1984. Both present pictures of the plants, their Russian and Latin names (and for the book in Kiev, Ukrainian names), the parts of the plants used, where they are grown or collected, the time of year to collect them, how to preserve them, the diseases and medical problems for which they are used, historical information and counterindications for their use. The illustrations in the second book are beautiful colored plates. The book discusses plants that help respiratory problems—resulting from colds and flu caused by coronaviruses or bacteria—as well as chronic respiratory problems such as asthma and emphysema, plants that treat skin infections—as well as auto-immune dermatological problems like eczema, and plants that treat diseases of the digestive system and other internal organs, the nervous system, and cardiac problems—some caused by viruses, bacteria, or allergies. The many émigrés who came from the Soviet Union to Denver, Colorado in the 1970s and 1980s were skilled in using plants for various diseases and medical problems because of shortages of factory-produced antibiotics and medicines in the Soviet Union.

Rebirth of Phytotherapy on a Sound, Scientific, Standardized Foundation

In the 1980s and 1990s, both Soviet citizens and émigrés from the USSR continued to self-medicate with medicinal plants. After the collapse of the Soviet Union in 1991, foreign pharmaceutical firms helped modernize former Soviet pharmaceutical firms. But, concomitantly, in the last decades of the 20th century, the emergence of bacteria and frightening "super bugs" resistant to antibiotics alerted specialists to the fact that use of medicinal plants–which had seemed backward in the past—was now innovative. Medicinal plants possess bactericide and immune-stimulating properties. Thus, Russian physicians and pharmacologists determined to standardize medicinal plants and plant products and emphasize the scientific basis and benefits of phytotherapy for both infectious and chronic diseases. Regional startups include "Parafarm" in Penza and other companies. Leaders of the movement in Moscow include Dr. Vladimir Korsun and his daughter Dr. Elena Korsun, Directors of the Institute of Phytotherapy in Moscow, who still dominate the field. They convene conferences, publish books, and publish a journal, *Prakticheskaya fitoterapiia* (Practical Phytotherapy).

For example, Practical Phytotherapy, 2018, 2, includes an article on Phytotherapy in HIV infections--Korsun, V. F., Korsun, E. V. Eremin, V. F., Boreko, "O perspective fitotherapii VICh-infektsii," An article in Practical Phytotherapy, 2016, 1, discusses The History of Herbal Medicine of the Astrakhan Region", detailing collecting, cultivation, and research into botanicals that began in the early 18th century in this former Mongol khanate. The article reveals that Astrakhan has more than 100 forms of medicinal plants, many specific to the southern latitudes. Although a third of the plants are poisonous, efficacious varieties in the south have a higher content of active ingredients and thus stronger influence on the constitution than comparable varieties in the north. Fifty individuals now work in a factory that has produced 180 botanical products. One of the products highlighted in the article is an immune-strengthening product "Immunoflan"—that could prove useful for protection against infectious diseases as well as chronic medical problems [105].

Six papers presented at a phytotherapy conference in January 2019 in the science city of Chernogolovka, near Moscow, dealt specifically with infectious diseases. These included grippe or influenza, Hepatitis B and C, HIV, infectious inflammations in women, pulmonaria, viral diseases, and herpetic diseases, such as shingles. These papers have been published in the Conference Proceedings, *Sovremennye problemy fitoterapii i travnichestva* (Contemporary Issues of Phytotherapy and Herbalism.) We cannot review these articles in this chapter but we do note that M. I. Gadzhiev *et al.* (five co-authors) discusses treating Hepatitis B and C with the seeds and fatty oil of Black tmin or caraway seeds—an ancient remedy that archeology has shown dates back 8,000 years and later to Egyptian King Tutankhamen and that was used by Russian researchers in previous centuries, as discussed above in this chapter. Records of five patients are presented to show efficacy. Boreko, E. I. *et al.* (three co-authors) discuss the efficacy of the lektins in nine plants—powder of the flowers of calendula, leaves of salvia, mint, Melissa, corn, St. John's Wort, and three others to inhibit the coronavirus causing seasonal flu. The article recommends the commercial preparation Хитокор (khitokor) as a prophylactic for flu presenting charts and scientific data as proof [106].

Finally, we briefly examine the regimens of the two therapists in Russia sent me in March 2020 to prevent COVID-19 and treat symptoms of this very contagious disease that do not require hospitalization. The phytotherapists have different training and live in very different regions of Russia. Dr. Elena Korsun is a physician living in Moscow. She and her father are directors of a Phytotherapy Institute at a university in Moscow. They are academics, publishing their research on phytotherapy for various diseases in articles and books that contain charts and tables, sophisticated terminology, and scientific testing. Dr. Korsun convenes conferences and teaches others. Mar'yam Murtuzaliva is a self-trained healer who practices in Dagestan in the Caucasus. The Caucasus is extremely heterogeneous ethnically and linguistically. Her patients are mainly non-Russian and, although Makhachkala, the capital of Dagestan, is a city, many of Mar'yam's patients are agriculturalists and animal herders. Thus, one of her specialties is eliminating parasites conveyed to humans by animals, wild and domesticated. With regard to COVID-19, both of these phytotherapists have used a similar approach. Both agree that cases where the virus has attacked the lungs and caused severe over-reaction call for hospitalization and ventilators. Nevertheless, it now appears that serious, lethal cases seem related to the elderly and those with compromised immune systems and occur only in a fraction of those testing positive. They are even more minuscule statistically in the general population. Indeed, most people contracting the virus are asymptomatic or have only mild cases. Thus, the two Russian phytotherapists both recommend that susceptible people stay out of crowds as much as possible and that they and others first and foremost strengthen their immune systems to ward off this coronavirus. They also recommend wearing masks to avoid the spread of contagion, good hygiene, and cleansing the nasal passages with saltwater or commercial salt-water products to prevent the entrance of the virus. For those with mild cases the two phytotherapists advocate isolation and self-quarantine to prevent spread to others. For treating the symptoms of mild cases both recommend plants served in decoctions, infusions and teas that have been proven effective in other coronavirus cases—head colds and influenza—to improve breathing and quell fevers and coughs.

The main difference between the two Russian phytotherapists in the last approach in that Dr. Korsun uses commercial products as well as plants whereas Mar'yam Murtuzaliva relies on combinations of plants crushed into a powder and diluted in boiled water, a procedure for which she provides detailed recipes. Building on successfully combatting SARS, Dr. Korsun first recommends FitoGor to strengthen the immune system. This product includes mint, melissa, calendula, salvia, St. John's Wort and other ingredients that have anti-viral properties. She recommends Propolis, made of pine sap, honeycomb and other ingredients to strengthen immunological reaction, strengthen phagocyte activity, stimulate lymphocytes, raise the antimicrobial activity of antibiotics and the bactericide properties of blood serum. She also recommends oil of *Nigella salvia L.* seed presented by one Mohammed Salah in the journal Immunopharmacology. Tantsetum is a commercial Russian product that strengthens immunity and is sold abroad. To prevent the virus from entering the nasal passages, Dr. Elena Korsun recommends using a home-made saline solution or Akva Maris with a sea-water base. For the treatment of symptoms of mild COVID-19, she recommends Akva Maris Plus that not only strengthens immunity but fights inflammation and improves breathing function. To treat symptoms of the virus she recommends chamomile, salvia, eucalyptus, and the commercial product Ingrafitol. She addresses mental health, depression, and anxiety from isolation suggesting serotonin, Ivan-Tea, chamomile, and the commercial product Farmatsvet [107].

Mar'yam Murtuzaliva gives recipes and regimens for plants. She first builds up the immune system with tansy (*Chrysanthemum tanacetum vulgarae*), artemisia (*Raphanan sativas L.*), carnation/cloves, barberry root, oil of Zhivitsa (which has a pine sap base), and other plants. To treat cough, breathing difficulties, and other symptoms of mild COVID-19, she provides recipes for decoctions made of medicinal plants—in addition to tansy, artemisia—the seeds of *Silybum marianum*, family *Asteraceae*, and many other plants. The only commercial product she uses is Propolis—made of honeycomb and other ingredients [108].

CONCLUSION

It is obvious that Russia is an example of "Herbal Medicine: Back to the Future" for the use of botanicals to prevent and treat the symptoms of infectious diseases as well as chronic medical problems. This does not mean that we can do away with antibiotics, chemically synthesized medicines, and chemotherapy for cancers. Russian phytotherapists and healers do not discount vaccines and antibiotics for treating infectious diseases. However, relying on centuries of empirical evidence, the successful restoration to health of their patients through application of parts of plants and certain commercial plant products is proof of the efficacy of certain botanicals in preventing infectious diseases, building up the immune system to counter infectious diseases, and treating the symptoms of infectious diseases.

CONFLICT OF INTEREST

The author declares that there is no conflict of interest in this chapter.

CONSENT FOR PUBLICATION

Not applicable.

ACKNOWLEDGEMENTS

Declared none.

REFERENCES

[1] Wilson Colin. Rasputin and the Fall of the Romanovs. Secaucus, N.J.: Citadel Press, 116.

[2] Schola Medica Salernitana," 8 pp, Wikipedia, The Medical School of Montpellier. https://en.wikipedia.org/wiki/Schola_Media_Salernitana

[3] Skliarova EK, Zharov LV, Depgousova TG. Istoriia farmatsiia. (History of Pharmacy). Rostov-on-Don: Feniks 2015; 95.

[4] Vernadsky G. Ancient Russia. New Haven and London: Yale University Press, 1964 and Vernadsky, G. Kievan Russia. New Haven: Yale University Press, 1959. For one source for archeological finds in current Kazakhstan and Russian connections with China and other cultures, see Akishev, K. and Akishev, A. The Ancient Gold of Kazakhstan. Alma-Ata: Oner, 1983, pp. 33-44.

[5] Skliarova, *et al.* Istoriia farmatsii, pp. 81-82.

[6] Moss WG. A History of Russia, Vol. I. London: Anthem Press, 2005. pp. 61-63, 83-84.

[7] Davies N. God's Playground: A History of Poland. Vol. 1. The Origins to 1795. New York: Columbia University Press, 1982. Subtelny, Orest. Ukraine A History. Toronto: Toronto University Press, 1994, pp. 123-177.

[8] De Madariaga, I. Russia in the Age of Catherine the Great. New Haven and London: Yale University Press, 1981, pp. 229-231, 308-313, 427-451.

[9] Russian Justice: The Short Version, cited in Dmytryshyn, Basil. Medieval Russia: A Source Book,

900-1700. Second Edition. New York: The Dryden press, 1973, pp. 44-50.

[10] Skliarova, Istoriia farmatsii, p. 82.

[11] Popov, G. Russkaia narodnaia meditsina, 1903," in "Belena, https://ru.wikipedia.org/wiki/Belena, p. 2 of 5. See also "Boligolov". https://re/wikipefia.org/wiki/bologolov

[12] Skliarova, Istoriia farmatsiia, p. 82.

[13] Conroy MS. Malaria in late Tsarist Russia. Bull Hist Med 1982; 56(1): 41-55. [PMID: 7046859]

[14] Skliarova, ibid., p. 82.

[15] Kotukov TN. Kul'tiviruemye i dikorastushchie lekarstvennye rasteniia: Spravochnik.Cultivated and wild medicinal plants: A Handbook. Kiev: Naukova dumka 1975; pp. 74-7.

[16] Kotukov, ibid., pp. 108-110.

[17] Kotukov, ibid., p. 135.

[18] Turova AD, Sapozhnikova RN. Lekarstvennye rasteniia SSSR i ikh primenenie. Medicinal plants of the USSR and their Application 1984; 148-50.

[19] Turova, et al., ibid., pp. 146-148.

[20] Hamilton GH. The Art and Architecture of Russia. New Haven: Yale University Press 1982; pp. 194-208.

[21] Salo V M. Istoriia farmatsiii v Rossii. History of Pharmacy in Russia 2007; 9-10.

[22] Salo, ibid., pp. 9-29.

[23] Skliarova, *et al,* Istoriia farmatsii, p. 147.

[24] Marks G, Beatty WK. Epidemics: The Story of Mankind's Most Lethal and Elusive Enemies from Ancient Times to the Present. New York: Charles Scribner's Sons 1976; pp. 72-91.

[25] Mirskii M, Bogoiavlenskii N. Meditsina drevnei Rusi.Medicine of Ancient Russia. Moscow: Rodina 2018; p. 265.

[26] Mirskii, ibid., p. 266.

[27] Mirskii, Ibid., p. 266-267.

[28] Mirskii, Ibid., 267-269.

[29] Wikipedia: Anthrax, Mirskii, ibid., 270. https://en.wikipedia.otrg/wiki/anthrax

[30] Russia Beyond the Headlines: The Siberian Plague, accessed May 5, 2020. http://www.rbth.com/longrreads/siberian_plague

[31] Alexander JT. Bubonic Plague in Early Modern Russia: Public Health and Urban disaster. Baltimore, London: The Johns Hopkins University Press 1980; p. 148.

[32] Alexander JT. Catherine the Great: Life and Legend. NY: Oxford University Press 1989; pp. 143-8.

[33] Conlon James M. The Historical Impact of Epidemic Typhus, pp. 11-12 on the internet.

[34] Gudienė V. The medical treatment of Maria, Dowager Empress of the Russian Empire: an analysis of her prescription book from 1807 and 1808. Pharmazie 2016; 71(11): 670-9. [PMID: 29441974]

[35] McGrew, Roderick. Russia and the Cholera: 1923-1932. Madison and Milwaukee, 1865, p. 146.

[36] McGrew, ibid., pp. 140-141.

[37] McGrew, ibid., p. 145.

[38] Salo V M. Istoriia farmatsii v Rossii, p. 76.

[39] Foust CM. Rhubarb: The Wondrous Drug. Princeton: Princeton University Press 1992. [http://dx.doi.org/10.1515/9781400862658]

[40] Alexander, Bubonic Plague, pp. 276-278.

[41] Conroy. M. S. In Health and In Sickness: Pharmacy, Pharmacists and the Pharmaceutical Industry in Late Imperial, Early Soviet Russia. Boulder, CO: East European Monographs, 1994, p. 139.

[42] Bolotov AA. Ekonomicheskii magazin, 1780, Part 2, No. 31, 78-79 cited in A. A. Utkin, A. F. Gammerman, V. A. Nevskii, Bibliografiia po lekarstvennym rasteniiam: (Bibliography on Medicinal Plants) [hereafter Utkin et al. Bibliografiia], Moscow: Academy of Sciences of the USSR, 1957, p. 70.

[43] Bolotov, "Lekarstva ot ponos" (Medicine against diarrhea), Ekonomicheskii magazin, 1780, part 1, no. 26, 405-408, in Utkin et al, Bibliografiia, p. 70, 8. For contemporary information: 1-5 and ,1-4. Accessed 29 June 2020. https://ru.wikipedia.org/wiki/Xvoshch https://ru.wikipedia.or/wiki/Zemeevik_bol'shoi

[44] Bolotov, "O nekotoyekh prostykh no s pol'zoi aprobirovannekh lekarstvakh," (About some simple, but useful medicines), Ekonomicheskii magazin, 1783, part 14, no. 33, 110-111. Cited in Utkin et al, Bibliografiia, p. 91, 34.

[45] Bolotov, "Nechto o komarakh" (A few things about mosquitoes), Ekonomicheskii magazine, 1783, part 15, no. 53, 15 cited in Utkin et al, Bibliografiia, p. 90. Modern research: Kesharvarz. A., Miniayan, M., Ghannadi, A., and Mahzouni, P, "Effects of *Carum carvi* L. (Caraway) extract and essential oil on TNBS-induced colitis in rats," Research in Pharmaceutical Sciences, 8, 1, 1-8 2013, 2.

[46] Lepekhin II. O domashnik sredstvakh prostym narodom v bolezniakh upotrebliaemykh" (About substances available at home used by the common people for diseases). St. Petersburg, 1792, cited in Utkin et al, Bibliograpfiia, p. 89, 121.

[47] Conroy MS. In Health and In Sickness, pp. 139-140.

[48] Conroy M S. In Health and In Sickness, On Malaria see Conroy, M. S. "Malaria in Late Tsarist Russia," Bulletin of the History of Medicine 1982; 56(1): 41-55.

[49] The book by Boplan (Beauplan) on medicine in Ukraine and by A. Levshin on the use of herbs for diseases amongst the Kirgiz-Kazakh people of the steppe.Utkin et al, Bibliografiia. 1832; pp. 128-9.

[50] Smel'skii E. Konvulsii u ditiati, prodolshavshiesia bolee trekh sytoki izlechennye...*Artemisia vulgaris*" (Convulsions among children lasting for more than three days treated [with] *Artemisia vulgaris*], Drug zdrava [Friend of Health], ...1835, cited in Utkin, Bibliografiia, p. 133. Modern information: "Facty Health: The total Body Benefits of Betaine, and Facty Health, The Necessity and Health Benefits of Choline. https://en.wikipedia.org/wiki/Artemisia_cina https;//facty.com/lifestyle/wekkness/the-total-body-benefits-of-betaine/? https;//facty.com/lifestyle/wellness/the-necessity -and health -benefits-of-choline/?

[51] Articles on Bird Cherry in Utkin, *et al,* Bibliografiia, pp. 137 1, 140 12 and 141 4. Article by Aleksandra Telichowska *et al,* in Nutrients 2020, 12, 1966, 7, 4, 5, 7, 8-11.

[52] Koren' sumbuly kak sredstva ot xolery," (The Roots of Sumbul as a substance against Cholera), Proceedings of the [Russian] Military Economic Society, cited in Ultkin, et al, Bibliografiia, p. 154, #15. https://ru.wikipedia.org/wiki/Ferula_muskusnaia. For medicinal uses, see Pharmacognosy Review, 2012, Jul-Dec 6 (12): 141-146. http://www.ncbi.rim. Nih.gov/pmc/articles/PMC3459456/

[53] Lavrent'ev S. Air ili iaver (Acorus calamus) ot likoradki , (Acorus calamus against fevers) Proceeding of the [Russian] Military Economic Society, cited in Utkin, Bibliografiia, p. 154, 17.

[54] Russian article cited in Utkin, Bibliografiia, p. 156, 6. Modern information.

[55] Russian article cited in Utkin, Bibliografiia, p. 157, 19 and 29. Modern information: "Jerusalem artichoke," Wikipedia. http;//en.wikipwdia.org/wiki/Jerusalem_artichoke

[56] Russian article cited in Utkin, Bibliografiia, p. 157, #30. On Boligolov see Wikipedia, ru.

Wikipedia.org./wiki/Boligolov and CAB International's very lengthy website.

[57] Conroy M S. Conroy, M. S., In Health and In Sickness, p. 141.

[58] Conroy, ibid., pp. 141-142.

[59] Dmitri Ivanovsky, Wikipedia https://en.wikipedia.org/wiki/Dmitri_Ivanovsky

[60] Andrei Famitsyn, Wikipedia https:// en.wikipedia.org/wiki/Andrei_Famitsyn

[61] Conroy MS. Women pharmacists in Russia before World War I: women's emancipation, feminism, professionalization, nationalism and class conflict," Women and Society in Russia and the Soviet Union, ed. Linda Edmondson. Cambridge University Press, 1992, 48-76. Discussion of Ol'ga Gabrilovich, 63-64. [http://dx.doi.org/10.1017/CBO9780511520877.005]

[62] Conroy, In Health and In Sickness, p. 161.

[63] Conroy, In Health and In Sickness, pp. 142-143.

[64] Conroy, In Health and In Sickness, pp. 137-161. Also, Conroy, M. S. The Soviet Pharmaceutical Business during Its First Two Decades, 1917-1937. Peter Lang, 2006., pp. 11-18. One source of information on the Russian chemical industry just before World War I is Khimicheskoe delo v Rossii (The Chemical Business in Russia) Odessa, 1913.

[65] Conroy, In Health and In Sickness, p. 161.

[66] Anikst Mikhail, Chernevich Elena. Russian Graphic Design, 1880-1917. See also: Preis-kurant tovarov firmenoi zadelki ...R. Keler i Ko v Moskve (Price -List of the Products of the Firm Produced by R. Keler and Company), Moscow, 1914 ; Optovyi Preis Kurant v ...Sklada Aptekarskikh tovarov Oskar Getling v Moskove. Firma sushchestvuet' v 1875 goda (Wholesale Price-list of the Warehouse of Pharmacy Products Oscar Getling in Moscow, a Firm established in 1875) n. d. but before 1917 as it sports the doble-headed eagle; Opyt istoricheskago ocherka Vozniknoveniia i Razvitiia vsego Aptekarskago Dela v Rossii a v chastnosti staroi Nikol'skoi apteki prinadlezhashchei nyne Tovarichestvu "V. K. Ferrein"...osnovannoi v 1701 godu (The Historical Outlines of the Rise and Development of Pharmaceutical Businesses in Russia , and in particular, the Old Nikol'skii Pharmacy, founded in 1701, now belonging to the Closely-Held Partnership V. K. Ferrein. Moscow, 1911.

[67] Conroy, In Health and In Sickness, pp. 320-348.

[68] Conroy, The Soviet Pharmaceutical Business, p. 20.

[69] Conroy, The Soviet Pharmaceutical Business, p. 20.

[70] Conroy, The Soviet Pharmaceutical Business, pp. 20-22.

[71] Conroy, In Health and In Sickness, pp. 39-56, 64-108.

[72] Conroy, In Health and In Sickness, pp. 64-76.

[73] Conroy, In Health and In Sickness, pp. 33-44, 54.

[74] Conroy, ibid., pp. 64-76.

[75] Conroy, In Health, pp. 57-64.

[76] Conroy, In Health and In Sickness, p. 42.

[77] Conroy, In Health and In Sickness, pp. 153-160, 162-174.

[78] Conroy M S. P. A. Stolypin, Marxists, and Liberals Versus Owners of Pharmacies and Pharmaceutical Firms in Late Imperial Russia," in Emerging Democracy in Late Imperial Russia. ed. Conroy, M. S. Boulder: University Press of Colorado, 1998, pp. 122-124.

[79] Conroy, In Health and In Sickness, pp. 320-348.

[80] Conroy, The Soviet Pharmaceutical Business, pp. 29-42.

[81] Conroy, The Soviet Pharmaceutical Business, pp. 48-49. Also, Joseph M. Conlon, "The Historical Impact of Epidemic Typhus, p. 15 and Frederick Holmes, Typhus on the Eastern Front, on the eastern front, 3pp. www.kums.edu/wwi/index-of-essays/typhus

[82] Conroy M S, Sosonkina VF. Conroy, Draft of article slated for the Hoover Digest, summer 2020, based on materials in the Hoover archive, Boxes 33, 147-148, 182, 184, and on materials from Belarusian archives.

[83] Bertrand Patenaude, The Big Show in Bololand. Stanford: Stanford University Press 2002.

[84] Seramumo_inf_ligoma_polyginimas_1925-1-28. Lithuanian statistics sent me by Dr. of Pharmacy and Pharmaceutical Historian Vilma Gudiene, Kaunas, Lithuania.

[85] Conroy, In Health and In Sickness, pp. 399-419 and Conroy, The Soviet Pharmaceutical Businesss, pp. 51-72.

[86] Sosonkina VF. Farmatsevticheskoe delo v Belarusi. (The Pharmaceutical Business in Belarus). Minsk, 2014, p. 88 and Sosonkina, V. F. Istoriia farmatsii Belarusi. (The History of Pharmacy in Belarus). Minsk, 2016. p. 38.

[87] For information on excessive exports see Conroy, The Soviet Pharmaceutical Business, pp. 201-210. For details on the other information in this paragraph and that preceding see Conroy, The Soviet Pharmaceutical Business, passim.

[88] Conroy, The Soviet Pharmaceutical Business, pp. 210-211.

[89] Information in this paragraph and the two preceding from Conroy, The Soviet Pharmaceutical Business, pp. 210-213.

[90] Conroy MS. Medicines for the Soviet Masses during World War II. Boulder, New York, Toronto: University Press of America 2008; pp. 45-74.

[91] Conroy, ibid., pp. 118-126.

[92] Conroy, ibid., pp. 110-112.

[93] Conroy, ibid., pp. 125, 159.

[94] Conroy, ibid., pp. 92-96.

[95] Conroy, Medicines for the Soviet Masses during World War II, p. 199.

[96] Conroy, The Soviet Pharmaceutical Business during Its First Two Decades, pp. 221-222.

[97] Conroy, Medicines for the Soviet Masses during World War II, p. 80.

[98] Conroy, Medicines for the Soviet Masses, pp. 82-85.

[99] Conroy, Medicines for the Soviet Masses, pp. 200-201.

[100] All information from reminiscences in the paragraphs above interviews published in Conroy, Medicines for the Soviet Masses, pp. 201-203.

[101] Conroy, Medicines for the Soviet Masses, pp. 204-208. The shipments may have been payment for lend-lease pharmaceuticals and equipment from the United States. The American Department of Commerce reports on the shipments do not give reasons for them.

[102] Conroy, Medicines for the Soviet Masses, p. 209.

[103] Sokhey SS. The Production of Pharmaceuticals in the Country. Indian J Pharm 1959; 21: 231-4.

[104] Conroy MS. The Soviet Pharmaceutical Industry and Dispensing, 1945-1953. Europe-Asia Studies, 978- 979.

[105] Isotoriia fitoterapii astakhanskoi oblasti," Prakticheskaia fitorerapiia, no. 1, 2016, pp. 6014.

[106] Sovremennye problemy fitoterapii i travnichestva: materialy V mezhdunarodugo c"ezda.

CHAPTER 4

Azadirachta Indica (Neem) in Various Infectious Diseases

Monica Joshi[1] and **Bala Prabhakar**[1,*]

[1] *Shobhaben Pratapbhai Patel School of Pharmacy & Technology Management, SVKM's NMIMS, Mumbai, Maharashtra, India*

Abstract: The 21st century is witnessing a war between mankind and microorganisms. The worldwide outbreak of infectious diseases is responsible for morbidity and mortality. The pharmaceutical industry has limited drugs in the pipeline against infectious diseases. Resistance of microorganisms against already available drugs is another concern. An initiative from researchers to search for new ways to prevent or treat infectious diseases is necessary. Many herbal drugs are known to be effective against pathogenic organisms from ancient times. Repurposing of herbal medicines for infectious diseases is a prodigious initiative. *Azadirachta indica,* commonly known as neem, is known to be effective against infectious diseases from ancient times. It is a member of the Meliaceae family. Leaves, seeds, fruits, and roots of this plant are reported to be effective according to Chinese, Ayurvedic, and Unani medicine. The plant has antiviral, antibacterial, and antifungal properties. The principal component of neem is azadirachtin. Other constituents, namely nimbolinin, nimbin, nimbidin, nimbidol, are also known to be having medicinal properties. Antibacterial and antifungal properties can be attributed to azadirachtin, quercetin, ß-sitosterol, gedunin, and polyphenolic flavonoids. Many pharmacological studies report antimicrobial efficacy of *Azadirachta indica.* The present chapter will explain the link between phytochemical constituents of neem to antimicrobial activity along with possible underlying mechanisms and pathways. Clinical studies on neem are also discussed in great detail to highlight the emergence of this traditional medicine into modern medicine in the battle against infectious diseases.

Keywords: Antibacterial, Antifungal, Antimalarial, Antiviral, *Azadirachta indica*, Azadirachtin, Meliaceae, Neem, Nimbin, Quercetin, Salannin.

INTRODUCTION

Microorganisms are creatures with a size range of few nanometers to 1000 micrometers. They are known to be present ubiquitously even inside the human

* **Corresponding author Dr. Bala Prabhakar:** Shobhaben Pratapbhai Patel School of Pharmacy & Technology Management, SVKM's NMIMS, Mumbai, Maharashtra, India; Tel/Fax: +91-022-42332000; E-mail: Bala.Prabhakar@nmims.edu

Ferid Murad, Atta-ur-Rahman, Ka Bian (Eds.)

body [1]. Some of them are referred to as beneficial microorganisms. Beneficial microorganisms help the plants by facilitating nitrogen fixation and affect the overall growth of plants [2]. Gut microflora is known to assist the digestion and total maintenance of the well-being of the human body [3]. The other class of microorganisms which cause harm by causing infectious diseases are pathogenic microorganisms [4]. Microorganisms from the class of bacteria, viruses, parasites, or fungi can be of pathogenic nature. The diseases caused by these pathogenic microorganisms are known as 'infectious diseases.' These diseases can be passed from one person to another *via* direct or indirect way [5]. Based on the intrinsic pathogenicity index (IPI), there can be three categories of pathogens, *i.e.*, low-level, high-level, and potential pathogens [6].

The modern era is fighting a war against pathogenic microorganisms which are evading our planet. According to the report issued by the World Health Organization (WHO) in 2016, 2-3 causes out of the list of top 10 global causes of deaths are infectious diseases like lower respiratory infections, diarrhoeal diseases, and tuberculosis. When the age group of less than 5 years is considered, around 6 causes out of the list of top 10 global causes of deaths are infectious diseases [7]. These results are alarming and indicating the morbidity and mortality rate because of infectious diseases. There is an emergence of many new infectious diseases which have turned into an epidemic or even pandemic. Chikungunya, Cholera, Ebola virus disease, Meningitis, Nipah virus infection, Zika virus infection, Coronavirus infections are some of the infections that have become epidemic or pandemic [8].

The main concern about the treatment of infectious diseases is the drug resistance developed by microorganisms. The drug discovery process is also largely affected by the phenomenon of drug resistance. It is observed that the rate of drug discovery has decelerated after the late 1960s mainly because of the fast drug resistance development compared to the much slower process of drug development [9].

Few researchers are strategically focussing on other ways to meet the need and supply correlation for antimicrobial therapy. The use of herbal medicines for the prevention and treatment of different diseases can be traced back to ancient times. Earlier, this use was predominantly restricted to underdeveloped or developing countries. The role of herbal medicine in the management of the SARS outbreak in 2003 has caught the attention of researchers across the globe. In the last few years, even developed countries are observed to believe in the use of herbal medicines. Herbal medicines can be used for the prevention or treatment of diseases and also as a supplement to allopathic medicines [10]. Repurposing of herbal medicines can also be an attractive strategy to combat many diseases [11].

Amongst many herbal medicines used for infectious diseases, this chapter focuses on the *Azadirachta indica* (Neem). The chapter will cover details about the plant and parts of the plant having phytoconstituents with pharmacological properties. This chapter also sheds light on the effective extraction of phytoconstituents from *Azadirachta indica* using optimum conditions to get maximum yield. A link between phytochemical constituents and their use in various infectious diseases is also discussed. Clinical studies giving strong evidence of the effectiveness of neem against infectious diseases are highlighted. The use of a nanoparticle approach for delivery of phytoconstituents of neem can give future direction for the best use of this plant.

AZADIRACHTA INDICA (NEEM)

Azadirachta indica belongs to the Meliaceae family. In Persian, "Azadi" means 'free' and "diracht" means 'tree.' The plant is named so because of its inherent insect-free properties [12]. It is commonly known as neem and also referred to as Indian lilac. Sub-humid to sub-arid climate is suitable for the growth of this evergreen plant [13]. The plant is mainly inhabited in Asian countries like India, Nepal, Pakistan, and Bangladesh [14]. Generally, the height of the plant is 30 meters, and the girth is 2.5 meters. The branches of the plant can spread across around 20 meters [15]. The leaves, seeds, fruits, flowers, bark, and roots, *i.e.*, almost the entire plant, are known to have medicinal properties [12]. Initially, the leaves are reddish-purple in colour, but the mature leaves look green in colour. The fruit of the plant has a smooth texture and ellipsoidal shape. It is greenish-yellow, to yellow in colour with the size of around 2 cm. The fruit contains sweet flesh and seeds [15]. Fig. (**1**) shows the leaves and fruits of the neem tree. Each part of the plant has unique properties which make it useful for different sorts of applications.

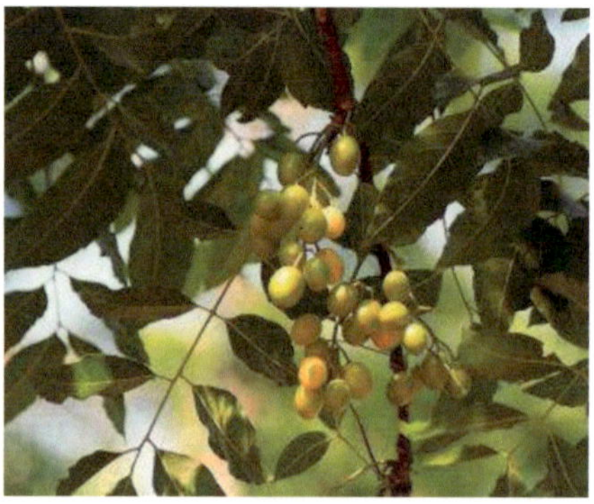

Fig. (1). Neem tree.

EXTRACTION

Different procedures can be employed for extracting various phytoconstituents from different parts of the plant. Saleh Al-Hashemi *et al.* have prepared neem leaf extract using the maceration method. Sample preparation prior to maceration was necessary to make the sample free from dust and foreign particles. The leaves were dried for 5 days, followed by grinding them into the powder. Maceration using methanol as a solvent was employed to prepare the crude extract of the dried powdered leaf sample. Defatting of the crude extract was done using water in order to remove lipids and other fatty substances. This water extract was further extracted with hexane, chloroform, ethyl acetate, and butanol. Different solvent extracts were obtained to analyse the solvent of choice for the extraction of antioxidants [16]. Santos, Klebson S. *et al.* showed that sequential pressurized liquid extraction of neem leaves was better compared to the ethanol extraction. Drying and milling prior to the extraction were done. The extraction pressure was adjusted at 100 bar with a temperature of 25 °C. The solvent flow rate was maintained at 1ml/min. After every extraction cycle, carbon dioxide was flushed through the system to remove the residual solvent from the previous step [17]. Voravuth Somsak *et al.* have dried the neem leaves using a hot air oven followed by a powdering step. The aqueous extract was prepared by boiling the dried powdered leaves in distilled water [18]. Tonthubthimthong, Pathumthip *et al.* have used CO_2 supercritical fluid extraction to extract nimbin from the neem seeds. The dried seeds were ground before extraction. The operating pressure, temperature, and flow rate for extraction were optimized at 23 MPa, 308 K, and 1.24 ml/min, respectively [19]. Shewale, Sandeep *et al.* have used stirred batch extraction of neem leaves for maximizing the phenolic compounds in neem extract. Before extraction, the leaves were dried in the shadow. The leaves were protected from sunlight so as to avoid the degradation of phenolic compounds. Hot air oven treatment was given, followed by grinding. The researchers showed that it is imperative to select an appropriate solvent for extraction for maximizing the yield of the desired bioactive phytoconstituents. Amongst the various solvents of different polarities, *i.e.*, methanol, ethanol, ethyl acetate, *n*-butanol, and water, 70% ethanol was optimized to be the solvent for maximum extraction of polyphenols. The use of water results in activation of polyphenol oxidase enzyme which is responsible for degradation of polyphenols giving extract with low polyphenol content. Another important aspect in extraction process is the ratio of solid to solvent. When the researchers increased the ratio from 1:10 to 1:50, there is increase in extraction of phenolic compounds. But after the ratio reaches 1:30, there is no substantial increase in extraction of phenols because of the lower concentration gradient compared to the lower ratios. Researchers observed an inverse relation between the particle sizes of the leaf powder and extraction efficiency of phenolic compounds. Lower-sized particles have higher exposed surface area to the extraction solvent resulting in more efficient extraction. But at the same time, the energy requirements for particle size reduction and separation efficiency have to be taken into consideration. Researchers showed that the batch agitated extraction method is an effective extraction technique compared to the one without agitation. Speed of agitation and extraction efficiency of total phenolic compounds from neem leaf powder share a positive correlation. Researchers optimized 300rpm agitation speed to get maximum extraction of polyphenols as a further increase in speed did not show a significant increase in the level of polyphenols. The effect of temperature on extraction efficiency of polyphenols from powdered neem leaves was also studied by researchers. As the temperature increases, the extraction increases due to an increase in extraction coefficient and overall solubility of phytoconstituents. But, high temperature might cause degradation of some of the phytoconstituents of the extract [20]. Liauw, Maria Yuliana *et al.* have extracted oil from neem seeds. The seeds were cleaned by washing with water and then dried. The dried seeds were powdered to increase the surface area to enhance the extraction efficiency. The extraction was carried out at different temperatures by the scientist to study its effect on the quality of the oil. Temperature increase adversely affects the oil quality. Saponification value, peroxide value, acid value, iodine value can be some of the markers used to determine the quality of the oil. Researchers stated that *n*-hexane was better suited for the extraction of oil from the neem seeds compared to the polar ethanol solvent [21]. Dai, Jianming *et al.* compared different extraction methods and different extraction conditions such as microwave irradiation (MAE), room temperature (RTE), and reflux (RFX) conditions for neem seed [22]. Johnson, Shaun *et al.* have compared supercritical carbon dioxide and supercritical carbon dioxide: methanol extraction. Total 100% of carbon dioxide was responsible for the extraction of nimbin and salanin. Introduction of carbon dioxide, methanol, for extraction is responsible for selective extraction of azadirachtin. A total of 20 and 6% methanol can be used for selective extraction of azadirachtin and nimbin, salannin respectively [23]. Table **1** enlists various extraction techniques and parameters involved in the extraction procedure.

Table 1. Extraction techniques and parameters for neem.

Extraction Technique	Part of the Plant	Sample	Solvent	Conditions	Purification	Ref.
Maceration	Leaf	Powder (140 g)	Methanol (260 ml)	3 days	Filtration and solvent evaporation under reduced pressure	[16]

(Table 1) cont.....

Extraction Technique	Part of the Plant	Sample	Solvent	Conditions	Purification	Ref.
Sequential pressurized liquid extraction	Leaf	Milled leaves (20 g)	*n*- hexane, ethyl acetate, water/ethanol (20:80 v/v) (60 ml)	60 min each	Solvent evaporation	[17]
Boiling	Leaf	Powder (1gm)	Distilled water (20ml)	6 hours	Filtration and vacuum evaporation	[18]
CO_2 supercritical fluid extraction	Seed	Powder (2gm)	Methanol (10ml)	-	-	[19]
Soxhlet extraction	Leaf	Powder (2gm)	Methanol ethyl acetate, ethanol, butanol, water (225ml)	-	-	[20]
Batch agitated extraction	Leaf	Powder (2gm)	Ethanol (60ml)	76 min	-	[20]
Solvent extraction	Seed	Powder (1:5)	*N*-Hexane, ethanol	3 hours	Centrifugation, filtration followed by evaporation	[21]
Microwave-Assisted	Seed	Powder (2 gm)	Petroleum ether (15 ml) followed by dichloromethane (15ml)	-	Filtration and solvent evaporation under reduced pressure	[22]
Microwave-Assisted Extraction	Seed	Powder (2 gm)	Methanol Followed by dichloromethane partition	-	Solvent evaporation under vacuum	[22]
Room Temperature Extraction	Seed	Powder (2 gm)	Petroleum ether (60 ml) followed by dichloromethane	12 hours	Solvent evaporation under vacuum	[22]
Room Temperature Extraction	Seed	Powder (2 gm)	Methanol (60 ml) followed by dichloromethane partition	-	Solvent evaporation under vacuum	[22]
Supercritical carbon dioxide extraction	Seeds	Coarse powder	Carbon dioxide, carbon dioxide:methanol	30 min	Evaporation	[23]

PHYTOCHEMICAL CONSTITUENTS

An array of phytochemical constituents is present in *Azadirachta indica.* The major classes of phytoconstituents can be enlisted as alkaloids, hydrocarbons, glycosides, phenolic compounds, and terpenoids [24]. Saleh Al-Hashemi *et al.* have studied the biochemical nature of neem leaf extract of different polarities. Hexane, chloroform, ethyl acetate, butanol, methanol, and water extracts were screened for analysing the presence of phytoconstituents of different classes. Except for triterpenoid and anthraquinone, flavonoids, saponins, steroids, alkaloids, amino acid, and tannins were found to be present in all six extracts [16]. Neem shows the presence of certain triterpenoids known as limonoids which are known to exhibit biological activities like insecticidal, antibacterial, antifungal, antimalarial, antiviral, and anticancer in humans [25]. A few important phytoconstituents of neem are azadirachtin, nimbin, nimbidin, nimbolinin, nimbidol, nimbanene, nimbandiol, nimbolide, and sodium nimbinate. Other phytoconstituents extracted from neem include gedunin, salannin, quercetin, ß-sitosterol, 6-desacetylnimbinene, ascorbic acid, *n*-hexacosanol and amino acid, 7-desacetyl-7- benzoylazadiradione, 7-desacetyl-7-benzoylgedunin, 17-hydroxya zadiradione, and nimbiol. Quercetin and polyphenolic flavonoids were also reported to be present in fresh neem leaves [14]. Details about a few important phytoconstituents of neem are presented below.

AZADIRACHTIN

IUPAC Name: Dimethyl (1*S*,4*S*,5*R*,6*S*,7*S*,8*R*,11*S*,12*R*,14*S*,15*R*)-12-acetylo-y-4,7-dihydroxy-6-[(1*S*,2*S*,6*S*,8*S*,9*R*,11*S*)-2-hydroxy-11-methyl-5,7,10-trioxatetra cyclo[6.3.1.$0^{2,6}$.$0^{9,11}$]dodec-3-en-9-yl]-6-methyl-14-[(*E*)-2-methylbut-2-enoyl]oxy -3,9-dioxatetracyclo[6.6.1.$0^{1,5}$.$0^{11,15}$]pentadecane-4,11-dicarboxylate.

Azadirachtin is also known as Aazadirachtin, Azadyrachtin, Bioneem, and Neemix. The structure of Azadirachtin is shown in Fig. (**2**). It is a microcrystalline yellow-green powder with a strong garlic odour [26]. It is the most important limonoid present in the neem. This active ingredient was extracted from the neem seed by David Morgan, and the structural determination was done after 17 years of discovery [27]. Researchers have proved the strong inhibitory effect of Azadirachtin on insect moulting and thus the overall growth of insects. But the positive side of this is nontoxic nature of azadirachtin to mammals. It has no adverse effect on non-target organisms and the environment. The reduced form of azadirachtin is known as dihydroazadirachtin. The insecticidal property of these two forms is similar. The toxicity data shows that dihydroazadirachtin shows low toxicity to mammals [28].

NIMBIN

IUPAC Name: methyl (1*S*,2*R*,3*R*,4*R*,8*R*,9*S*,10*R*,13*R*,15*R*)-2-acetyloxy-13-(f-ran-3-yl)-9-(2-methoxy-2-oxoethyl)-4,8,10,12-tetramethyl-7-oxo-16 oxatetracyclo [8.6.0.$0^{3,8}$.$0^{11,15}$]hexadeca-5,11-diene-4-carboxylate [29].

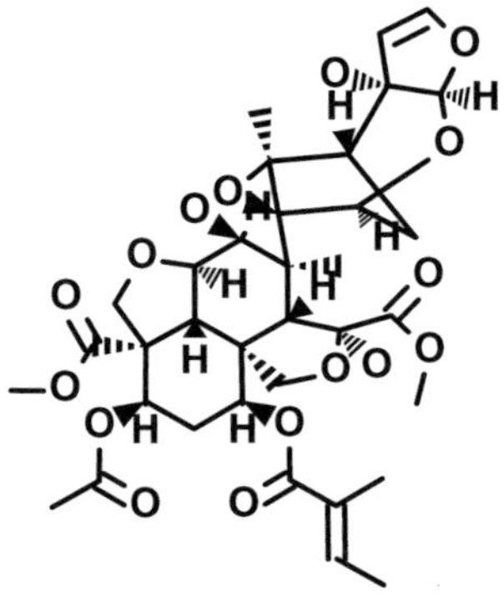

Fig. (2). Structure of azadirachtin.

Nimbin is another triterpenoid present in extracts of neem seeds [30]. The structure of the nimbin is shown in Fig. (**3**). It is reported to be effective in the treatment of arthritis, hypoglycaemia, peptic ulcers and also has anti-pyretic and antibiotic activity. Tonthubthimthong, Pathumthip *et al.* have extracted 0.18 mg of nimbin per gram of neem seed in one hour using supercritical CO_2 extraction [19].

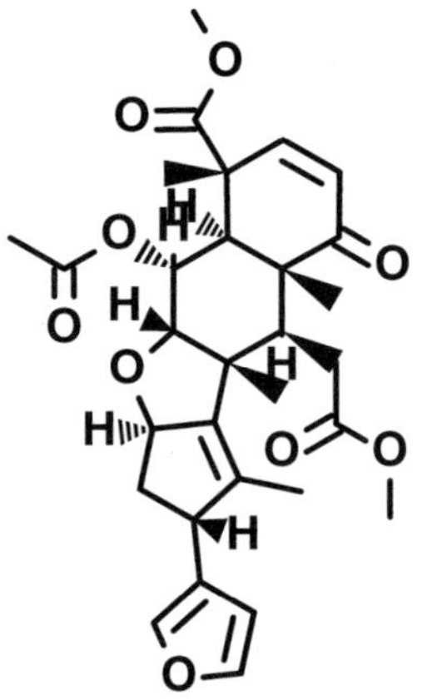

Fig. (3). Structure of nimbin.

SALANNIN

IUPAC Name: [(1*R*,2*S*,4*R*,6*R*,9*R*,10*R*,11*R*,12*S*,14*R*,15*R*,18*R*)-14-acetylox--6-(furan-3-yl)-10-(2-methoxy-2-oxoethyl)-7,9,11,15-tetramethyl-3,17-dioxapenta cyclo[9.6.1.$0^{2,9}$.$0^{4,8}$.$0^{15,18}$]octadec-7-en-12-yl] (*E*)-2-methylbut-2-enoate [31].

Salannin belongs to the limonoid class and is another important phytoconstituent present in neem. It is also reported to have insecticidal properties. Chemically, it is an acetate ester and a member of the furan class [31]. The structure of salannin is shown in Fig. (**4**). Researchers have stated that salannin is a bitter component of neem. It shows protective activity against gastric lesions. It also shows antibacterial activity against gram +ve and gram –ve bacteria. It also showed spermicidal activity against human spermatozoa [32].

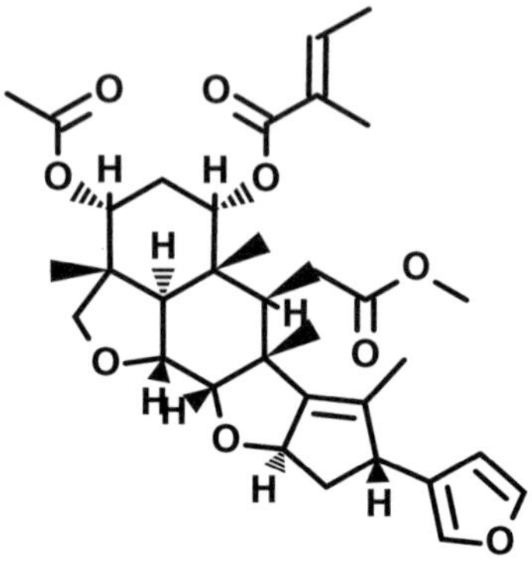

Fig. (4). Structure of Salannin.

CHARACTERIZATION OF PHYTOCONSTITUENTS OF NEEM

Characterization of macromorphological and micromorphological properties of the plant parts can help in the identification and differentiation at the genetic level. Researchers studied the macromorphological and micromorphological characteristics of leaves, fruits, seeds, stem, and bark of *Azadirachta indica* and *Melia* Azadirachta because the latter is occasionally misidentified with neem. DNA fingerprinting further helped in differentiating between the two plants by characterizing at the genetic level [33]. Characterization of the extract is a very crucial step that determines the phytoconstituents present in the extract. Researchers have developed a colorimetric method for the determination of the content of azadirachtin-related limonoids (AZRL) in the extracts of seed kernels of neem. The method involves the use of acidified vanillin solution in methanol. This solution is used for the colorization of standard azadirachtin or extracts of neem kernel. Various factors such as vanillin concentration, acid concentration, colour formation time, optimum conditions can be employed to achieve good detection and linearity [34]. In another study, researchers have isolated azadiramide A, a limonoid alkaloid, from neem seeds. The structural elucidation of the isolated compound was done by extensive spectroscopic analysis and quantum chemical calculation [35]. In another study, GC/MS analysis of an *n*-Hexane extract of leaves of *Azadirachta indica* identified 45 bioactive compounds. The antifungal activity of these compounds was analysed. Out of 45 compounds, 33 compounds showed antifungal activity [36]. Hossain, Mohammad

A. *et al.* have characterized the phytoconstituents of the crude extracts of neem by employing gas chromatography-mass spectrometry (GC-MS). The main advantage of using the modern technique for the characterization of phytoconstituents is its sensitivity. The GC-MS study proved that the compounds identified in the neem extracts contain hydrocarbons, phenolic compounds, terpenoids, alkaloids, and glycosides. Based on the GC-MS analysis, the selection of appropriate crude extract can be made to obtain the desired bioactive compounds [37]. In one study, high-performance thin-layer chromatography (HPTLC) fingerprinting of methanol extract and ethyl acetate subfraction of neem leaves was performed. HPTLC fingerprint of the methanol extract exhibited 16 peaks (Rf values between 0.03 and 0.96), whereas ethyl acetate subfraction showed 18 peaks (Rf values between 0.03 and 0.95). This technique can be successfully used for the analysis of genetic variability in different plant species [38]. In another study, researchers have tried bioassay-guided purification to characterize a diterpenoid compound, nimbidiol, present in the methanolic extract of the root and stem-bark of neem tree [39]. A group of scientists has characterized Azadirachtun extracted from the ethanolic extract of neem leaves. Thin-layer chromatography (TLC) was used for qualitative analysis of the phytoconstituent, whereas the quantitative analysis was performed using the high-pressure liquid chromatography (HPLC) technique [40]. Among different known phytoconstituents of neem, the azadirachtin class has been exploited for the commercial perspective. The other two phytoconstituents, namely, salanin and nimbin have a great potential for product development. The variation in nimbin and salanin content in neem trees from different provenances and even between the trees from one provenance was analysed by RP-analytical HPLC [41]. One report mentions the use of Fourier transform infrared spectroscopy (FTIR) and partial-least-square (PLS) multivariate regression analysis methods for analysing adulteration in neem oil, including adulterants like edible vegetable oil or extra virgin olive oil. The adulterants can cause potential health implications to consumers. The developed model was simple and accurate to validate the % composition of adulterated neem oil sample by following accurate analytical protocol. This model has special application in quality control of neem oil [42].

ROLE OF *AZADIRACHTA INDICA* (NEEM) IN VARIOUS INFECTIOUS DISEASES

Neem extract and phytoconstituents of neem are known to play a role against microorganisms like bacteria, viruses, and fungi. Though the exact mechanism of action of neem is ambiguous, the possible mechanism of antimicrobial action is through inhibition of microbial growth and breakdown of bacterial cell wall [14].

ANTIBACTERIAL ACTIVITY

The use of neem against various bacterial infections is widespread. A study was performed to evaluate the activity of neem extract against *Vibrio cholerae*, a bacterium that is known to cause infectious diseases like cholera and diarrhea. The methanol extract of neem leaf showed significant antibacterial activity against multi-drug resistant form of *Vibrio cholerae* (of serotypes O1, O139, and non-O-1, non-O139). The minimum inhibitory concentration (MIC_{90}) and minimum bactericidal concentration for the extract were noted to be >5 and 10 mg/ml, respectively [43]. In another study, the mechanism of antibacterial activity of neem nanoemulsion was studied by the membrane integrity and cell damage assessment of the bacteria, Vibrio vulnificus. The treated bacteria were found to release 85.3%, whereas the control sample released only 12.6% of the cytoplasmic material. The scanning electron microscopic analysis revealed that the bacterial cells treated with the neem nanoemulsion had disrupted and disintegrated cell walls, whereas the untreated bacterial cells possessed an intact cell wall. This study pointed out the possible mechanism of the neem against bacteria by causing physical damage, *i.e.*, disruption and release of cytoplasmic content [44]. The mechanism by which the bacterial growth is inhibited is mainly the breakdown of the bacterial cell wall [45].

ANTIVIRAL ACTIVITY

In one study, researchers isolated two polysaccharides from the leaves of *Azadirachta indica*. The derivatives of these polysaccharides were prepared chemically. The activity of these compounds against poliovirus type 1 was determined by employing a plaque reduction assay. The polysaccharides and their sulphated derivatives showed significant antiviral activity. The polysaccharides showed better antiviral activity compared to the sulphated derivatives. The mechanism of action of antiviral effect is by inhibition of viral replication at the initial stage [46]. In another study, the antiviral activity of methanolic extract fraction of neem (NCL-11) was thoroughly studied against the Coxsackie B group of viruses. The results suggested that a variety of compounds present in NCL-11 apart from flavonoids, triterpenoids and glycosides possess antiviral activity against Coxsackie B group of viruses. The virucidal effect of the fraction was maximum against coxsackievirus B-4. Its fraction showed interference at an early stage of virus replication [47]. The effect of aqueous extract of the neem bark against the Herpes simplex virus (HSV-1) was analysed, and the mechanistic insight was given. The entry of HSV-1 into the target cells was blocked after the treatment with the extract. The viral fusion was hampered by inhibiting HSV-1 glycoprotein-mediated cell-cell fusion and polykaryocytes formation [48]. In one report, the inhibitory activity of aqueous extract of neem leaves and Azadirachtin on Dengue virus type-2 was reported. *In vitro* antiviral assessment of extract was tested in $C_{6/36}$ cells by using virus inhibition assay. *In vivo* activity of the neem extract against Dengue virus type-2 in suckling mice was proved by inhibition of the virus replication. The treated mice showed an absence of clinical symptoms associated with Dengue. RT-PCR study also showed the absence of a 511 bp amplicon specific to the virus. The activity of neem extract against Dengue virus was evident from the study, whereas pure Azadirachtin was not effective against the virus, as proved by both *in vitro* and *in vivo* studies [49]. A study reported a possible mechanism of action by which acetone-water neem leaf extract showed antimicrobial activity. It was observed that the adhesion of erythrocytes which are infected with malarial parasites, to the endothelial cells is inhibited. The extract was reported to possess antiretroviral activity on account of inhibition of cytoadhesion [50].

ANTIFUNGAL ACTIVITY

In a study, the leaf oil of neem was analysed to test its activity against various fungal strains such as F. oxysporum, *A. flavus*, *A. fumigates*, *A. niger* , *C. albicans*, *Cladosporium* sp. *etc.* The antifungal activity was found to be dependent on the protein and carbohydrate contents of the oil. The contents of protein and carbohydrate in the oil had a direct relationship with the antimicrobial potential [51]. In another study, the effect of aqueous, ethanolic, and ethyl acetate extracts of neem leaves against the growth of some human pathogens like *Aspergillus flavus, Aspergillus fumigatus, Aspergillus niger, Aspergillus terreus, Candida albicans*, and *Microsporum gypseum* was tested *in vitro*. The fungal inhibitory activity showed a gradual increase with the concentration of the extract. The 20% ethyl acetate extract showed the strongest inhibitory activity compared to the other extracts.

High-Performance Liquid Chromatography (HPLC) and Nuclear Magnetic Resonance (NMR) spectroscopic analysis confirmed the presence of nimonol in the ethyl acetate extract. The ethyl acetate extract in the absence of nimonol exhibited reduced antifungal activity. But the isolated nimonol did not exhibit antifungal activity [52]. De Rezende Ramos, Alessandra *et al.* established the mechanistic effect of neem extract against *C. albicans*. Neem extract was shown to affect the surface hydrophobicity giving an anti-adhesive effect leading to the inhibition of *C. albicans* colonization [53].

ANTIMALARIAL ACTIVITY

A study by one group of scientists evaluated the transmission-blocking potential of NeemAzal® (an Azadirachtin enriched extract of neem seeds) using the rodent malaria *in vivo* model *Plasmodium berghei*/*Anopheles stephensi*. At an azadirachtin dose of 50 mg/kg mouse weight, NeemAzal® blocked the development of the vector totally [54]. In another study, the effect of methanolic extract of seed kernel of ripe and unripe fruits of neem on the erythrocytic proliferation of malaria parasite *Plasmodium berghei* strain ANKA was analysed. The study proved that the activity depends on the strain of the mouse undergoing treatment as well as the ripening stage of the neem fruit. The unripe fruit seed kernel showed substantial activity compared to the ripe fruit [55]. An acetone-water extract of neem leaves was found to inhibit malarial parasites in both forms *i.e.*, asexual form (trophozoites or schizonts) and sexual form (gametocytes). Thus, the neem leaf extract was found to be useful for the treatment of malarial infection as well as for the prevention of transmission of the infection *via* gametocytes [56].

TOXICOLOGICAL STUDY OF NEEM

A thorough analysis of toxicity is very important and a must in the case of natural products meant for the treatment of various diseases. The studies about the toxicity profile of extracts and a few phytoconstituents of *Azadirachta indica* are carried out by some researchers to establish a safe dose. In a study, the toxicity of ethanol extract of stem bark of neem was analysed by giving different doses (50, 100, 200 and 300 mg/kg) to Wistar rats *via* the oral route. Few biochemical parameters were unaltered, whereas other parameters showed a significant change. This suggested that the given doses of ethanolic extract of neem might not be completely safe for oral administration [57]. In another study, acute and 28-days subacute toxicological evaluation of neem oil were done. The acute toxicity analysis obtained the LD_{50} values to be 31.95 g/kg. The results of subacute toxicity evaluation showed that there was no change in feed, water, body weight, and biochemical parameters at the dose of 1600 mg/kg/day, proving it to be safe at this dose [58]. Another group of researchers has subjected azadirachtin to subchronic toxicity analysis in rats. Azadirachtin technical 12% was administered orally to male and female rats at doses of 500, 1000, and 1500 mg/kg/day for 90 days. There were no signs of toxicity, mortality, changes in tissue weight, pathology, and serum and blood parameters after the treatment period. The highest dose used for the analysis was also found to be safe [59].

CLINICAL STUDIES ON NEEM

The effectiveness of the neem extract and phytoconstituents isolated from the neem can be confirmed by clinical studies. A clinical study was done to analyse the antimicrobial effectiveness of neem extract dental gel on the oral cavity and compared it with a mouthwash containing chlorhexidine gluconate (0.2% w/v). The decrease in the salivary bacterial (*Streptococcus mutans* and *Lactobacilli* species) count was tested. The results showed that the reduction in the plaque index and the bacterial count was significantly higher in the neem extract gel group compared to the control group [60]. In another study, the safety and effect of acetone-water extract of neem leaf were tested on CD4+ cells in 60 HIV/AIDS patients. The CD4+ cell count was found to be improved. Other parameters such as body weight, haemoglobin count, and differential lymphocyte count were also reported to be improved. The extract was found to be safe and have a significant effect on CD4+ cells in HIV/AIDS patients [61]. In a study, researchers have investigated the efficacy of one spermicidal fraction isolated from neem oil, *i.e.*, NIM-76, against some bacteria, fungi, and polio virus. NIM-76 exhibited inhibitory activity against *Escherichia coli* and *Klebsiella pneumonia* in contrast to the whole neem oil. It also showed strong antifungal activity confirmed by the protective effect on mice having systemic candidiasis infection. The study concluded that NIM-76 exhibited strong, broad-spectrum anti-microbial activity when compared to the whole neem oil [62].

NANOFORMULATIONS OF NEEM

The use of nanotechnology to design a formulation of herbal extracts or phytoconstituents has gained popularity in the last few decades. There are numerous advantages offered by nanotechnology to improve the delivery of the phytoconstituents to the target site as well as the manifestation of therapeutic effect. In one study, oil in water (O/W) nanoemulsion of neem was formulated using neem oil Tween 20 and water. High-energy ultrasonication was used for the preparation of nanoemulsion. The neem nanoemulsion showed excellent activity against *Vibrio vulnificus*. Cell viability analysis proved that the nanoemulsion was non-toxic at the lower concentrations whereas it was toxic at higher concentrations [44]. In another study, poly(ε-caprolactone) nanocapsules loaded with neem oil were prepared. The emulsion-solvent evaporation method was used for the preparation of nanoformulation. The mean particle size of nanocapsules was around 400nm with a polydispersity index lesser than 0.2. Cytotoxicity and genotoxicity studied revealed an increase in toxic effect of neem formulations containing oleic acid [63]. In one study, the biosynthesis of silver nanoparticles was done using extract of neem leaves. The process is environmentally friendly because of the use of neem extract. The use of the extract is thought to provide a synergistic antibacterial effect with silver nanoparticles [64]. Another nanoformulation strategy employed solid lipid nanoparticles loaded with neem oil to treat acne and improve skin elasticity. The double emulsification method was used with the use of lecithin and Tween 80 for the preparation of solid lipid nanoparticles with a mean particle size of 221.6 ± 2.0 nm having excellent entrapment efficiency of 82.10%. The obtained nanoparticles were stable for around 3 weeks. The nanoformulation exhibited satisfactory activity against acne microbes and exhibited sustained effect [65]. One report compared the activity and toxicity of neem oil with a nanoemulsion loaded with neem oil. Tween 20 was used as a surfactant for preparing a nanoemulsion. The study proved that the antioxidant activity of neem oil was similar to that of nanoemulsion loaded with neem oil. But the cytotoxicity of neem oil on Hep-2 cells was reduced after loading it into a nanoemulsion [66].

CONCLUSION

Infectious diseases have been responsible for creating many hurdles into the path of human progress. Microbial resistance to the existing drugs and having a small amount of antimicrobial drugs in a pipeline warrant extensive research for the treatment of infectious diseases. The use of herbal drugs for the treatment of infectious diseases can be a rational approach. Neem is one such herbal drug known to have good efficacy against infectious diseases. The phytoconstituents of neem like azadirachtin, nimbin, salannin are also known to be having medicinal properties.

Neem is known to have antiviral, antibacterial, antifungal, and antimalarial properties. Thus, neem-based phytochemicals can be developed for treating infectious diseases by a systematic pre-clinical and clinical approach.

CONSENT FOR PUBLICATION

Not applicable.

CONFLICT OF INTEREST

The authors declare no conflict of interest, financial or otherwise.

ACKNOWLEDGEMENTS

Declared none.

REFERENCES

[1] Batt CA. Microorganisms.Reference Module in Food Science. Ithaca, NY, USA: Elsevier 2016; pp. 8-9.

[2] Raaijmakers JM, Paulitz TC, Steinberg C, Alabouvette C, Moënne-Loccoz Y. The rhizosphere: A playground and battlefield for soilborne pathogens and beneficial microorganisms. Plant Soil 2009; 321(1-2): 341-61.
[http://dx.doi.org/10.1007/s11104-008-9568-6]

[3] Neish AS. Microbes in gastrointestinal health and disease. Gastroenterology 2009; 136(1): 65-80.
[http://dx.doi.org/10.1053/j.gastro.2008.10.080]

[4] Yoo SM, Lee SY. Optical biosensors for the detection of pathogenic microorganisms. Trends in biotechnology 2016; 34(1): 7-25.

[http://dx.doi.org/10.1016/j.tibtech.2015.09.012]

[5] WHO. Health topics 2020. https://www.who.int/topics/infectious_diseases/en/

[6] De La Cal MA, Cerdà E, Abella A, Garcia-Hierro P. Classification of microorganisms according to their pathogenicity.InInfection Control in the Intensive Care Unit. Springer, Milano 2011; pp. 29-40.

[7] WHO. Causes of death, by WHO region 2020. https://www.who.int/gho/mortality_burden_disease/causes_death/top_10/en/

[8] WHO. Disease outbreaks 2021. https://www.who.int/emergencies/ diseases/en/

[9] Song YG. The history of antimicrobial drug development and the current situation. Vol. 44. Infect Chemother 2012; 263-8.
[http://dx.doi.org/10.3947/ic.2012.44.4.263]

[10] Wachtel-Galor S, Benzie IFF. 1 Herbal Medicine.Lester Packer, Ph D. 2011; 28: p. 1.

[11] Lim DW, Kim H, Kim YM, Chin YW, Park WH, Kim JE. Drug repurposing in alternative medicine: herbal digestive Sochehwan exerts multifaceted effects against metabolic syndrome. Sci Rep 2019; 9(1): 9055.
[http://dx.doi.org/10.1038/s41598-019-45099-x] [PMID: 31227732]

[12] Subapriya R, Nagini S. Medicinal properties of neem leaves: a review. Curr Med Chem Anticancer Agents 2005; 5(2): 149-6.
[http://dx.doi.org/10.2174/1568011053174828] [PMID: 15777222]

[13] Schmutterer H. Properties and Potential of Natural Pesticides from the Neem Tree, *Azadirachta Indica.* Annu Rev Entomol 1990; 35(1): 271-97.http://www.ncbi.nlm.nih.gov/ pubmed/2405771

[14] Alzohairy MA. Therapeutics role of *Azadirachta indica* (neem) and their active constituents in diseases prevention and treatment. Evid Based Complement Alternat Med 2016; 2016

[15] National Research Council (US) Panel on. The tree. Neem: A Tree For Solving Global Problems. US: National Academies Press 1992.

[16] Saleh Al-Hashemi ZS, Hossain MA. Biological activities of different neem leaf crude extracts used locally in Ayurvedic medicine. Pacific Science Review A: Natural Science and Engineering 2016; 18(2): 128-31.
[http://dx.doi.org/10.1016/j.psra.2016.09.013]

[17] Santos KS, Barbosa AM, Freitas V, *et al.* Antiproliferative activity of neem leaf extracts obtained by a sequential pressurized liquid extraction. Pharmaceuticals (Basel) 2018; 11(3): E76.
[http://dx.doi.org/10.3390/ph11030076] [PMID: 30061479]

[18] Somsak V, Chachiyo S, Jaihan U, Nakinchat S. Protective Effect of Aqueous Crude Extract of Neem (*Azadirachta indica*) Leaves on *Plasmodium berghei*-Induced Renal Damage in Mice. J Trop Med 2015; 2015: 961205.
[http://dx.doi.org/10.1155/2015/961205] [PMID: 26379714]

[19] Tonthubthimthong P, Chuaprasert S, Douglas P, Luewisutthichat W. Supercritical CO_2 extraction of nimbin from neem seeds - an experimental study. J Food Eng 2001; 47(4): 289-93.
[http://dx.doi.org/10.1016/S0260-8774(00)00131-X]

[20] Shewale S, Rathod VK. Extraction of total phenolic content from *Azadirachta indica* or (neem) leaves: Kinetics study. Prep Biochem Biotechnol 2018; 48(4): 312-20.
[http://dx.doi.org/10.1080/10826068.2018.1431784] [PMID: 29424626]

[21] Liauw MY, Natan FA, Widiyanti P. Extraction of neem oil (*Azadirachta indica* A. Juss) using n-hexane and ethanol: studies of oil quality, kinetic and thermodynamic. ARPN Journal of Engineering and Applied Sciences 2008; 3(3): 49-54.

[22] Dai J, Yaylayan VA, Raghavan GSV, Parè JR. Extraction and colorimetric determination of azadirachtin-related limonoids in neem seed kernel. J Agric Food Chem 1999; 47(9): 3738-42.

[http://dx.doi.org/10.1021/jf990227h] [PMID: 10552715]

[23] Johnson S, Morgan ED. Supercritical fluid extraction of oil and triterpenoids from Neem seeds. Phytochem Anal 1997; 8(5): 228-32. [http://dx.doi.org/10.1002/(SICI)1099-1565(199709/10)8:5<228::AID-PCA367>3.0.CO;2-C]

[24] Hossain MA, Al-Toubi WAS, Weli AM, Al-Riyami QA, Al-Sabahi JN. Phytochemical analysis and Antibacterial properties of *Azadirachta indica* (Neem) leaves extract against *E. coli*. Journal of Pharmacognosy and Phytochemistry 2013; 7(4): 1368-71. https://www.sciencedirect.com/science/article/pii/S1658365513000423

[25] Roy A, Saraf S. Limonoids: overview of significant bioactive triterpenes distributed in plants kingdom. Biological and Pharmaceutical Bulletin 2006; 29(2): 191-201.http://www.ncbi.nlm.nih.gov/pubmed/16462017

[26] PubChem. Bethesda (MD): National Library of Medicine (US), National Center for Biotechnology Information; 2004-. PubChem Compound Summary for CID 5281303, Azadirachtin 2021. https://pubchem.ncbi.nlm.nih.gov/compound/Azadirachtin#section=IUPAC-Name

[27] Mordue(Luntz) AJ. Azadirachtin from the neem tree *Azadirachta indica*: its action against insects. Anais da Sociedade Entomológica do Brasil 2000; 29(4): 615-32. http://www.scielo.br/scielo.php?script=sci_arttext&pid=S0301-80592000000400001&lng=en&nrm=iso&tlng=en

[28] Gonzalez-Coloma A, Reina M, Diaz CE, Fraga BM, Santana-Meridas O. Natural product-based biopesticides for insect control. In: Liu H, Mander L, Eds. Comprehensive Natural Products II 2010; 237-68.https://www.sciencedirect.com/topics/agricultural-and-biological-sciences/azadirachtin

[29] PubChem. Bethesda (MD): National Library of Medicine (US), National Center for Biotechnology Information; 2004-. PubChem Compound Summary for CID 108058, Nimbin 2021.https://pubchem.ncbi.nlm.nih.gov/compound/Nimbin#section=Computed-Properties

[30] Jarvis AP, Johnson S, David Morgan E, Simmonds MSJ, Blaney WM. Photooxidation of nimbin and salannin, tetranortriterpenoids from the neem tree (*Azadirachta indica*). Journal of chemical ecology 1997; 23(12): 2841-60.https://link.springer.com/article/10.1023/A:1022523329255

[31] PubChem. Bethesda (MD): National Library of Medicine (US), National Center for Biotechnology Information; 2004-. PubChem Compound Summary for CID 6437066, Salannin 2021. https://pubchem.ncbi.nlm.nih.gov/ compound/Salannin

[32] MADHU DC, Nair GR. Antiulcer, antibacterial and spermicidal activities of salannin. Indian drugs 2001; 38(12): 629-32. https://www.academia.edu/16526883/Anti_ulcer_Anti_bacterial_and_Spermicidal_activities_of_salannin_Indian_Drugs_38_12_2001_629_632

[33] El-Hawary SS, El-Tantawy ME, Rabeh MA, Badr WK. DNA fingerprinting and botanical study of *Azadirachta indica* A. Juss. (neem) family Meliaceae. Beni-Suef Univ J Basic Appl Sci 2013; 2(1): 1-13. [http://dx.doi.org/10.1016/j.bjbas.2013.09.001]

[34] Dai J, Yaylayan VA, Raghavan GSV, Parè JR. Extraction and colorimetric determination of azadirachtin-related limonoids in neem seed kernel. Journal of agricultural and food chemistry 1999; 47(9): 3738-42.https://pubs.acs.org/doi/pdf/10.1021/jf990227h

[35] Zhu J, Lu X, Fan X, Wu R, Diao H, Yu R, *et al.* A new cytotoxic salannin-class limonoid alkaloid from seeds of *Azadirachta indica* A. Juss. Chin Chem Lett 2018; 29(8): 1261-3. [http://dx.doi.org/10.1016/j.cclet.2017.11.042]

[36] Akpuaka A, Ekwenchi MM, Dashak DA, Dildar A. Biological activities of characterized isolates of n-hexane extract of *Azadirachta indica* A. Juss (Neem) leaves Nature and Science 2013; 11(5): 141-7.http://www.sciencepub.net/naturehttp://www.sciencepub.net/nature.21

[37] Hossain MA, Al-Toubi WAS, Weli AM, Al-Riyami QA, Al-Sabahi JN. Identification and characterization of chemical compounds in different crude extracts from leaves of Omani neem.

Journal of Taibah University for Science 2013; 7(4): 181-8. https://www.tandfonline.com/doi/full/10.1016/j.jtusci.2013.05.003

[38] Dalal S, Seasotiya L, Bai S, Bharti P, Malik A, Taneja R. Preliminary Phytochemical Evaluation and HPTLC Fingerprinting of Leaves of *Azadirachta indica*. American Research Journal of Biosciences 2015; 1: 42-7.www.arjonline.org

[39] Mukherjee A, Sengupta S. Characterization of nimbidiol as a potent intestinal disaccharidase and glucoamylase inhibitor present in *Azadirachta indica* (neem) useful for the treatment of diabetes. Journal of enzyme inhibition and medicinal chemistry 2013; 28(5): 900-10. https://www.tandfonline.com/doi/full/10.3109/14756366.2012.694877

[40] Soni H, Mishra K, Sharma S, Singhai AK. Characterization of Azadirachtin from ethanolic extract of leaves of *Azadirachta indica*. Journal of Pharmacy Research 2012; 5(1): 199-201. https://www.cabdirect.org/globalhealth/abstract/20123162616

[41] Sidhu OP, Kumar V, Behl HM. Variability in triterpenoids (nimbin and salanin) composition of neem among different provenances of India. Industrial Crops and Products 2004; 19(1): 69-75.https://www.infona.pl//resource/bwmeta1.element.elsevier-4e40c6e7-03a0-3-41-bdce-eae1523dbea9

[42] Elzey B, Pollard D, Fakayode SO. Determination of adulterated neem and flaxseed oil compositions by FTIR spectroscopy and multivariate regression analysis. Food Control 2016; 68: 303-9. [http://dx.doi.org/10.1016/j.foodcont.2016.04.008]

[43] Thakurta P, Bhowmik P, Mukherjee S, Hajra TK, Patra A, Bag PK. Antibacterial, antisecretory and antihemorrhagic activity of *Azadirachta indica* used to treat cholera and diarrhea in India. J Ethnopharmacol 2007; 111(3): 607-12. [http://dx.doi.org/10.1016/j.jep.2007.01.022] [PMID: 17314018]

[44] Jerobin J, Makwana P, Suresh Kumar RS, Sundaramoorthy R, Mukherjee A, Chandrasekaran N. Antibacterial activity of neem nanoemulsion and its toxicity assessment on human lymphocytes *in vitro*. International journal of nanomedicine 2015; 10(Suppl 1): 77.

[45] Tiwari R, Verma AK, Chakraborty S, Dhama K, Singh SV. Neem (*Azadirachta indica*) and its potential for safeguarding health of animals and humans: A Review. Vol. 14. J Biol Sci 2014; 110-23. [http://dx.doi.org/10.3923/jbs.2014.110.123]

[46] Faccin-Galhardi LC, Yamamoto KA, Ray S, Ray B, Carvalho Linhares RE, Nozawa C. The *in vitro* antiviral property of *Azadirachta indica* polysaccharides for poliovirus. J Ethnopharmacol 2012; 142(1): 86-90. [http://dx.doi.org/10.1016/j.jep.2012.04.018] [PMID: 22855945]

[47] Badam L, Joshi SP, Bedekar SS. *In vitro* antiviral activity of neem (*Azadirachta indica*. A. Juss) leaf extract against group B coxsackieviruses. The Journal of communicable diseases 1999; 31(2): 79-90.https://europepmc.org/article/med/10810594

[48] Tiwari V, Darmani NA, Yue BYJT, Shukla D. *In vitro* antiviral activity of neem (*Azardirachta indica* L.) bark extract against herpes simplex virus type-1 infection. Phytotherapy Research 2010; 24(8): 1132-40.http://doi.wiley.com/10.1002/ptr.3085

[49] Parida MM, Upadhyay C, Pandya G, Jana AM. Inhibitory potential of neem (*Azadirachta indica* Juss) leaves on dengue virus type-2 replication. J Ethnopharmacol 2002; 79(2): 273-8. [http://dx.doi.org/10.1016/S0378-8741(01)00395-6] [PMID: 11801392]

[50] Udeinya I, Mbah A, Chijioke C, Shu E. An antimalarial extract from neem leaves is antiretroviral. Transactions of the Royal Society of Tropical Medicine and Hygiene 2004; 98(7): 435-7.https://academic.oup.com/trstmh/article-lookup/doi/10.1016/j.trstmh.2003.10.016 [http://dx.doi.org/10.1016/j.trstmh.2003.10.016]

[51] Asif M. Antimicrobial potential of *Azadirachta indica* against pathogenic bacteria and fungi. Journal of Pharmacognosy and phytochemistry 2012; 1(4): 78-83.

[52] Mahmoud DA, Hassanein NM, Youssef KA, Abou Zeid MA. Antifungal activity of different neem leaf extracts and the nimonol against some important human pathogens. Brazilian Journal of Microbiology 2011; 42(3): 1007-6. http://www.scielo.br/scielo.php? script=sci_arttext&pid=S1517-83822011000300021&lng=en&nrm=iso&tlng=en [http://dx.doi.org/10.1590/S1517-83822011000300021]

[53] de Rezende Ramos A, Lüdke Falcão L, Salviano Barbosa G, Helena Marcellino L, Silvano Gander E. Neem (*Azadirachta indica* a. Juss) components: Candidates for the control of Crinipellis perniciosa and Phytophthora ssp. Microbiological research 2007; 162(3): 238-43. https://pubmed.ncbi.nlm.nih.gov/16872817/

[54] Lucantoni L, Yerbanga RS, Lupidi G, Pasqualini L, Esposito F, Habluetzel A. Transmission blocking activity of a standardized neem (*Azadirachta indica*) seed extract on the rodent malaria parasite *Plasmodium berghei* in its vector Anopheles stephensi. Malaria journal 2010; 9(1): 1-0. https://link.springer.com/articles/10.1186/1475-2875-9-66

[55] Habluetzel A, Pinto B, Tapanelli S, Nkouangang J, Saviozzi M, Chianese G, *et al.* Effects of *Azadirachta indica* seed kernel extracts on early erythrocytic schizogony of *Plasmodium berghei* and pro-inflammatory response in inbred mice. Malaria journal 2019; 18(1): 1-9. https://malariajournal.biomedcentral.com/articles/10.1186/s12936-019-2671-8 [http://dx.doi.org/10.1186/s12936-019-2671-8]

[56] Udeinya JI, Shu EN, Quakyi I, Ajayi FO. An antimalarial neem leaf extract has both schizonticidal and gametocytocidal activities. American journal of therapeutics 2008; 15(2): 108-. http://journals.lww.com/00045391-200803000-00004 [http://dx.doi.org/10.1097/MJT.0b013e31804c6d1d]

[57] Ashafa AOT, Orekoya LO, Yakubu MT. Toxicity profile of ethanolic extract of *Azadirachta indica* stem bark in male Wistar rats. Asian Pac J Trop Biomed 2012; 2(10): 811-7. [http://dx.doi.org/10.1016/S2221-1691(12)60234-2] [PMID: 23569852]

[58] Deng YX, Cao M, Shi DX, *et al.* Toxicological evaluation of neem (*Azadirachta indica*) oil: acute and subacute toxicity. Environmental toxicology and pharmacology 2013; 35(2): 240-6.

[59] Raizada RB, Srivastava MK, Kaushal RA, Singh RP. Azadirachtin, a neem biopesticide: subchronic toxicity assessment in rats. Food Chem Toxicol 2001; 39(5): 477-83. [http://dx.doi.org/10.1016/S0278-6915(00)00153-8] [PMID: 11313114]

[60] Pai MR, Acharya LD, Udupa N. Evaluation of antiplaque activity of *Azadirachta indica* leaf extract gel--a 6-week clinical study. J Ethnopharmacol 2004; 90(1): 99-103. [http://dx.doi.org/10.1016/j.jep.2003.09.035] [PMID: 14698516]

[61] Mbah AU, Udeinya IJ, Shu EN, Chijioke CP, Nubila T, Udeinya F, *et al.* Fractionated neem leaf extract is safe and increases CD4+ cell levels in HIV/AIDS patients. American journal of therapeutics 2007; 14(4): 369-74. http://journals.lww.com/00045391-200707000-00011

[62] SaiRam M, Ilavazhagan G, Sharma SK, *et al.* Anti-microbial activity of a new vaginal contraceptive NIM-76 from neem oil (*Azadirachta indica*). J Ethnopharmacol 2000; 71(3): 377-82. [http://dx.doi.org/10.1016/S0378-8741(99)00211-1] [PMID: 10940573]

[63] Pasquoto-Stigliani T, Campos EVR, Oliveira JL, Silva CMG, Bilesky-José N, Guilger M, *et al.* Nanocapsules containing neem (*Azadirachta indica*) oil: development, characterization, and toxicity evaluation. Scientific reports 2017; 7(1): 1-2.www.nature.com/scientificreports/

[64] Tripathi A, Chandrasekaran N, Raichur AM, Mukherjee A. Antibacterial applications of silver nanoparticles synthesized by aqueous extract of *Azadirachta indica* (Neem) leaves. J Biomed Nanotechnol 2009; 5(1): 93-8. [http://dx.doi.org/10.1166/jbn.2009.038] [PMID: 20055111]

[65] Vijayan V, Aafreen S, Sakthivel S, Reddy KR. Formulation and characterization of solid lipid nanoparticles loaded Neem oil for topical treatment of acne. J Acute Dis 2013; 2(4): 282-6.

[http://dx.doi.org/10.1016/S2221-6189(13)60144-4]

[66] Rinaldi F, Hanieh PN, Longhi C, Carradori S, Secci D, Zengin G, *et al.* Neem oil nanoemulsions: characterisation and antioxidant activity. Journal of enzyme inhibition and medicinal chemistry 2017; 32(1): 1265-73. https://www.tandfonline.com/doi/full/10.1080/14756366.2017.1378190

CHAPTER 5

Contribution of Novel Delivery Systems in the Development of Phytotherapeutics

Rabab Kamel[1,*]

[1] *Pharmaceutical Technology Department, National Research Centre, El-Bohooth Street, Cairo, Egypt*

Abstract:
Background: Since ancient times, herbal medicine has been widely used worldwide. The advancement of pharmaceutical technology and pharmacotherapy has allowed the great expansion in the development of novel drug delivery systems.

Purpose: The use of these novel delivery systems has remarkable advantages over conventional ones including: improved drug solubility, bioavailability, biological effect, and stability, in addition to improved toxicological profile and decreased side effects. Most natural products suffer from low solubility, low bioavailability, instability, difficult administration, and unpleasant odor and taste leading to low compliance, which limits its use.

Methods: The exploration of novel drug carriers to incorporate plant actives and extracts can improve their use and administration producing a revolution in the pharmaceutical and cosmeceutical fields for the prevention as well as treatment of several diseases including infectious diseases. Different types of nanometric and micrometric delivery systems can be used; these comprise lipid-based, polymer-based, polysaccharide-based, surfactant-based, and cholesterol-based systems and nanoemulsions in addition to hybrid nanoparticles.

Conclusion: The present article focuses on the role of the novel carriers in the development and revival of herbal medicine. The types, composition, efficacy, and challenges of different new carriers are discussed.

Keywords: Efficacy, Herbal, Nanoparticles, Pharmacotherapy, Solubility.

INTRODUCTION

Since the existence of human civilization, herbal remedies have been widely used for treatment and prophylaxis. They represent an important section of ancient culture in countries such as India, China, and Egypt [1]. The use of herbal pro-

* **Corresponding author Rabab Kamel:** Pharmaceutical Technology Department, National Research Centre, El-Bohooth Street, Cairo, Egypt; Tel: 00201113639193; E-mail: drrababk@hotmail.com

Ferid Murad, Atta-ur-Rahman, Ka Bian (Eds.)

ducts has been recognized by physicians as well as patients for their high therapeutic value. Besides their therapeutic potential, herbs have been used as disease preventors, cosmetics, and dietary supplements and for reducing obesity. Traditional medicine was highly propagated especially in developing countries for its availability and low cost. According to the World Health Organization, a great portion of the population in developing countries reaching 80% relies on traditional medicine for health care purposes [2]. The ability of herbal medicines to treat a wide variety of diseases with low cost and minor side effects is an important advantage [3]. Therefore, the evolution of phytotherapy has attracted a great portion of researchers.

Phytotherapeutics is a great section in the pharmaceutical industry. The global market of medicines deriving from herbal origin increased from 18 billion $ in 2005 to 26 billion $ in 2011 and is expected to expand to 111 billion $ by the end of 2023. This great expansion may be because many plant-derived products are delivered as dietary supplements and nutraceuticals. Around fifty percent of the drugs which were approved between 1981 and 2006 were, directly or indirectly, derived from natural products [1].

Much effort has been devoted for the development of novel carriers for herbal products aiming to improve the solubility of the active ingredient, ameliorate the physical and chemical stability, minimize the degradation process, reduce any toxicity, mask any bad or bitter taste, decrease the dose as well as the frequency of administration, and improve the biological effect [4]. Novel phytotherapeutics must, therefore, increase patient compliance.

NOVEL HERBAL DRUG DELIVERY SYSTEMS

Enormous efforts and investigations are necessary to prepare a suitable herbal delivery system because of many difficulties linked to physicochemical properties, physiological factors, and validation processes. The complexity of herbal extract, the presence of multiple active agents, different sources of the herbs, undetermined dosage regimen, and the need for advanced assay procedures are the main problems faced.

This concept appears to be challenging although several nano-carriers for herbal extracts have been investigated and have fulfilled efficiency comparable to that of chemically synthesized drugs.

The novel delivery systems must deliver the active entity to the site of action at the required dose and time. However, this is facing great challenges. A great proportion of the biologically active constituents of derived from plants are highly water-soluble, but has a low bioavailability, because they are unable to cross lipid membranes, in addition to their high molecular sizes, which result in their low efficacy. Others have low-water solubility with hydrophobic nature, which results in low absorption and bioavailability, and increased systemic clearance, which needs repeated administration or increased dose. Some herbal products have succeeded to show good activity *in vitro* but failed to attain good results *in vivo*. On the other hand, some components of herbal extracts are incompatible with other ingredients used in the formulation, which limit their use [5, 6]. Also, the chemical complexity of extracts is an additional challenge faced by researchers during the preparation, characterization, and evaluation of the formulations. Scientific advances can solve these problematic aspects. An ideal drug delivery system must be able to control drug release, in other words, it can modulate the pharmacokinetics and pharmacodynamics of the active agent by achieving the required changes in absorption, distribution, and elimination, which therefore can improve product efficacy and safety [3]. For example, the literature reported the improved multi-functional efficacy of naturally-derived drugs like Rutin [7 - 10, 11 - 15], Diosmin [16, 17, 18 - 20], Curcumin [21 - 26], and Resveratrol [27, 29 - 33] using nano-encapsulation to overcome their low aqueous solubility. Different types of formulated herbal novel preparations are discussed in this literature.

SCAFFOLDS

Scaffolds are an architectural matrix used in tissue engineering to replace or facilitate the growth of damaged or diseased tissues using biomaterials. They can provide controlled drug delivery and stimulate tissue growth. The drug release kinetics from the scaffold is dependent on the structure and porosity of the scaffold. Different polymers can be used in the preparation of the scaffolds; these can be classified into: natural polymers (alginate, collagen, chitosan, and gelatin) and synthetic polymers (polyacrylates, polyamides). Generally, a combination of physically or chemically crosslinked polymers can also be used [34]. The lipophilic tetrandrine is an alkaloid isolated from *Stephania tetrandra,* it has multiple biological functions like the reduction of blood pressure, anti-inflammatory, immunosuppressive, scavenger of free radicals, and it can be used in liver diseases and tissue regeneration. Controlled release porous chitosan-gelatin scaffolds loaded with tetrandrine were prepared to sustain the drug release [35].

Another study used nanofibrous scaffolds composed of poly-lactic acid and coated by aloe vera gel for wound dressing [36]. *Equisetum arvense* extract and nanohydroxyapatite were loaded into PLA solution to fabricate composite nanofibrous scaffolds for bone tissue engineering [37]. *Hemigraphis alternata* extract was incorporated into the chitosan scaffold for infectious wounds [38]. A herbal scaffold including *Cissus quadrangularis extract* with natural biopolymers alginate and *O*-carboxymethyl chitosan had an osteoinductive effect [39]. A 3D scaffold composed of poly-lactic acid loaded with baicalin showed high bone formation potential [40]. An antibacterial nanofibrous mat was fabricated by electrospinning and loaded with crude bark extract of *Tecomella undulate* for wound healing [41]. Nanofibrous scaffolds containing a combination of hydroxyapatite and *Cissus quadrangularis* showed a synergistic osteogenic effect [42]. Also, an electrospun scaffold was developed using biodegradable polymer and an old herbal drug for wound healing, complete biodegradation of the prepared patch was proved and confirmed its green nature [43]. All these studies showed that scaffolds are a good approach to deliver active herbal moiety for tissue engineering.

NOVEL DRUG DELIVERY SYSTEMS BASED ON NANOTECHNOLOGY

Nanotechnological advances have increasing applications in the pharmaceutical industry and research areas. These can provide many advantages including the enhancement of the solubility and stability of active constituents, extending the biological effect, improving the absorption and adjustment of the degree of hydrophilicity/lipophilicity. This technology can also be used to control the distribution of the active ingredient aiming to target specific tissues or organs [2, 44].

Nano-science has a great role in the advancement and development of biomedical fields; however, some challenges are present for example complexity and high cost of some preparation materials and procedures, difficulty of scaling up and irreproducibility. On another side, nanoparticles may have certain risk factors to the health and environment due to their tiny particle size allowing their inhalation and penetration through the biological membranes, which can cause many un-preferred side effects and diseases.

Several nanotechnology-based approaches can be exploited for the preparation of various types of nanocarriers. The main types of nano-phytotherapeutics discussed in the literature are listed below.

Polymer-Based Nanoparticles

Polymer-based nanoparticles have special advantages such as the ability to solubilize hydrophobic drugs, improve the passage through biological membranes, dose reduction, drug targeting [45], stability, and non-toxicity [46].

Polymers can be classified according to their source into natural, semi-synthetic, and synthetic polymers, and according to their chemical structure polymers can be categorized into nonionic, anionic, and cationic polymers [47] Fig. (**1**). Polymers derived from natural sources like alginate, chitosan, and pectin are generally available at low prices, biocompatible, bioadhesive, safe, and eco-friendly.

Poly (DL-lactic acid) nanoparticles encapsulating triptolide were prepared to overcome the problems of poor solubility and toxicity of the drug. The produced nanoparticles were spherical with a smooth surface [48]. Camptothecin for intravenous administration was loaded in modified chitosan nanoparticles for tumor targeting and better stability [49].

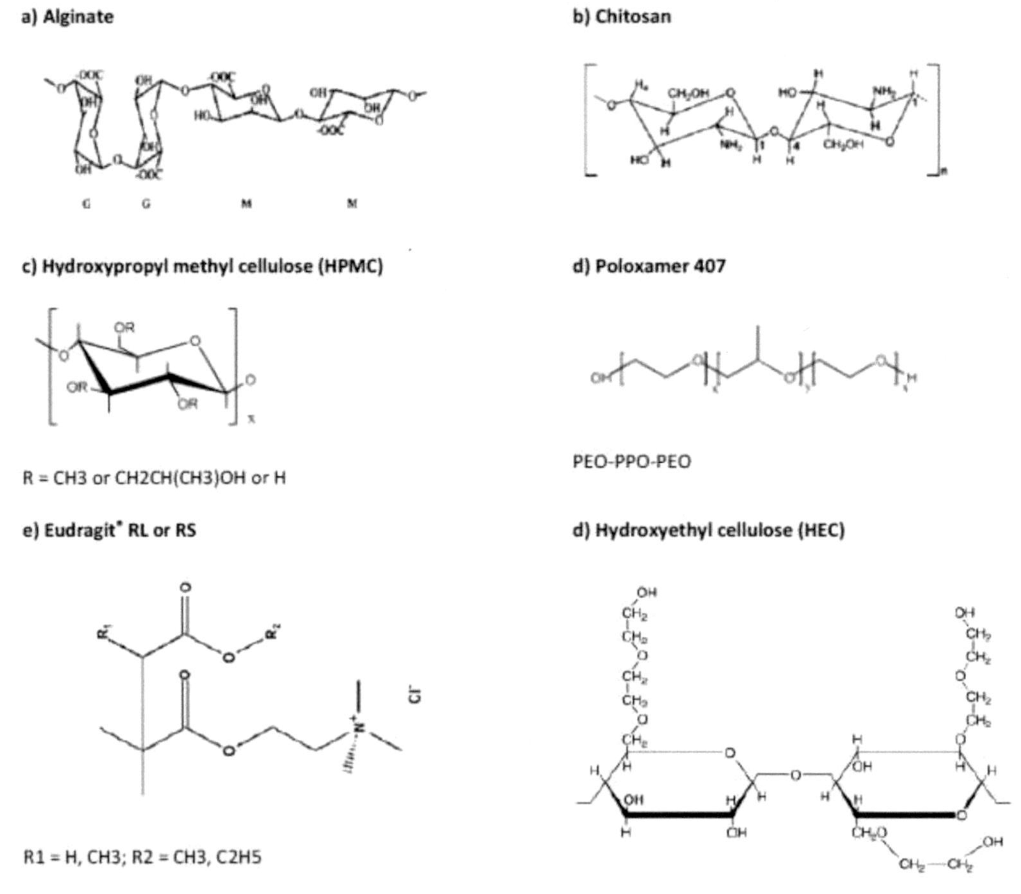

(Fig. 1) contd.....

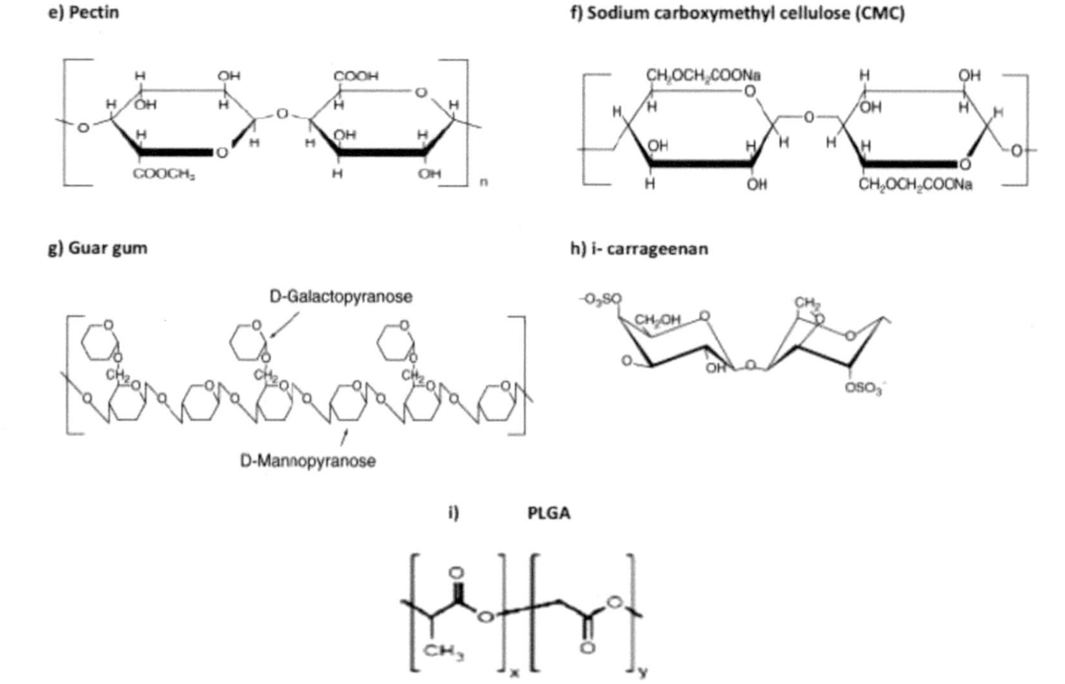

Fig. (1). Chemical structure of some polymers used for the preparation of various novel drug delivery systems.

To overcome the problems related to the low solubility of hypericin, an injectable suspension of polymeric nanoparticles was developed for the drug using the biodegradable and biocompatible polymers polylactic acid (PLA) and polylactic-co-glycolic acid (PLGA), which facilitated the systemic drug use for the early diagnosis of cancer [50]. Catechin-loaded chitosan nanoparticles were prepared to improve its antioxidant effect [51]. Also, the immunomodulatory activity of the extract of *Ziziphus mauritiana* was improved by using chitosan nanoparticles [52]. Quercetin polymeric nanoparticles were prepared to improve its absorption [53].

The extracts of leaves of *Ocimum sanctum* were loaded into sodium alginate chitosan nanoparticles and demonstrated a better and long-lasting antimicrobial activity [54]. Also, Garlic oil was encapsulated into chitosan nanoparticles which had a rod-shape and was found to have a significantly higher curing effect against induced neurotoxicity compared to plain Garlic oil [55].

Curcumin is a hydrophobic polyphenolic compound, extracted from rhizomes of *Curcuma longa,* and is characterized by its versatile biological effects. The preparation of polymeric nanoparticles has been one of the novel methods used to solve its bioavailability problems. *N*-isopropylacrylamide, *N*-vinyl-2-pyrrolidone, and poly(ethylene glycol) monoacrylate cross-linked copolymers were used to prepare curcumin-loaded nanoparticles which showed high activity against pancreatic cancer [56]. Curcumin-loaded PLGA nanospheres were prepared using a solid/oil/water emulsion solvent evaporation method and showed high efficacy against prostate carcinoma [57]. In another study, the prepared nano-sized formulation (2- 40 nm) enhanced the antimicrobial activity of curcumin [58].

The Chinese medicinal plant *Magnolia officinalis* containing Honokiol as an active ingredient with anti-inflammatory, antithrombotic, antirheumatic, antioxidant, and anxiolytic properties was loaded in polymeric nanoparticles which overcame its hydrophobicity and facilitated its vascular administration [59]. The preparation of polymeric nanocapsules containing coumarin enhanced its bioavailability and anti-tumor effect by improving its solubility [60]. The antibacterial, antifungal, and antiviral properties of *Harungana madagascariensis* extract were improved by incorporation into poly(D,L-lactide-co-glycolide) (PLG) nanoparticles [61].

Quercetin is a natural flavonoid having multiple pharmacological effects, such as anti-inflammatory, antitumor, antiviral, inhibitory of cataracts in diabetics, antihistaminic, in addition to cardiovascular, antioxidant, and hepatoprotective effects. Quercetin nanoparticles were prepared by the nanoprecipitation technique using Eudragit® E and polyvinyl alcohol (PVA). The nanoparticles attained higher anti-superoxide formation, superoxide anion scavenging, and anti-lipid peroxidation activities than Quercetin itself [62].

LIPID-BASED NANOPARTICLES

Lipid-based nanoparticles have been developed since 1990. They consist of a lipid, an aqueous phase, and a suitable surfactant. They have many advantages such as protection of sensitive drugs from chemical and physical degradation and extended drug release [63]. They can be prepared by hot or cold homogenization Fig. (**2**). According to drug distribution with the nanoparticles, three models are present, namely, homogeneous, drug-enriched shell, and drug-enriched core [64].

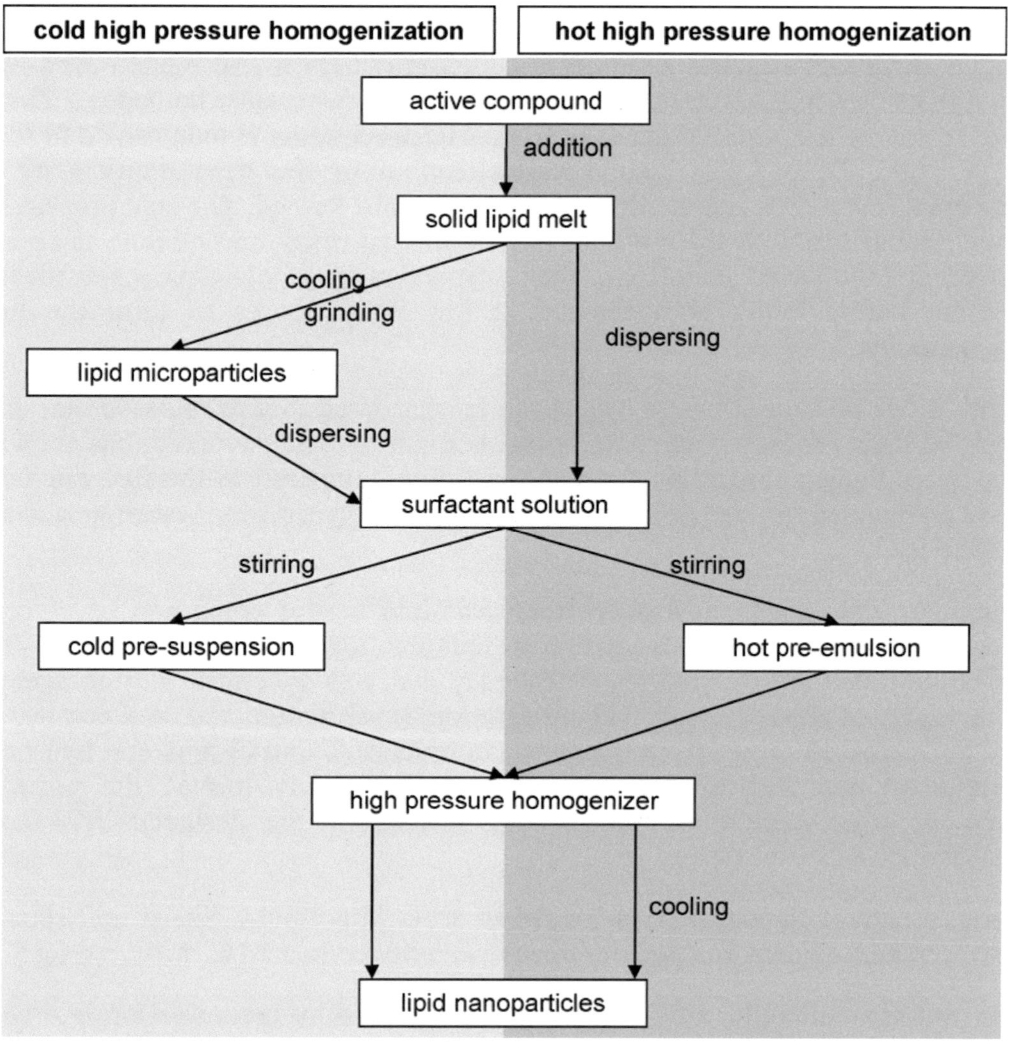

Fig. (2). Difference between the cold and hot high-pressure homogenization techniques.

A new generation of lipid nano-carriers has been developed to overcome the drawbacks of the 'old' generation. The new generation consists of lipid/oil mixture, which allows for higher drug loading and lower risk of drug expulsion out of the matrix [64, 65].

Literature has described many methods for the preparation of this type of colloidal carriers; however, the high-pressure homogenization (HPH) technique has many advantages compared to others, including: possible scaling up, minimal use of organic solvents, and short production time. Therefore, it is industrially feasible. Fig. (**2**) shows the difference between the hot and cold HPH techniques [63]. In the case of the hot HPH, the drug is uniformly dispersed in the molten lipid. The heated surfactant aqueous solution is added gradually to the melted drug-lipid mixture using a high shear mixing device. Then, high-pressure homogenization is used to reduce the particle size as desired. The preparation is then cooled to room temperature. During this step, recrystallization of the lipid droplets in the nanoemulsion occurs and the lipid nanoparticles are formed. The cold process has some similarities with the hot one, but the molten drug-lipid mixture is rapidly cooled and subjected to milling, then suspended in a cold aqueous surfactant solution before being homogenized at low temperatures to form the lipid nanoparticles.

Many drugs of natural origin have been encapsulated in a lipid-based carrier to improve their efficacy. Quercetin, a plant-origin natural flavonoid, has shown a five times higher absorption from the intestine compared to the free quercetin when formulated in solid lipid nanoparticles using glyceryl monostearate and soy lecithin [66].

Quercetin was loaded in a nanostructured lipid carrier composed of glyceryl monostearate, stearic acid, and soy lecithin for topical application. The preparation had high entrapment efficiency and was spherical with an average particle size of about 200 nm. The preparation showed promoted drug permeation and an increased drug amount retained in epidermis and dermis and had good antioxidant and anti-inflammatory effects. This study proved the potential targeting effect with a prolonged drug release by the designed lipid-based transdermal delivery system [67].

Rutin, a natural flavonoid, was loaded in a lipoid colloidal carrier and showed enhanced anti-oxidant and photoprotective activity compared to the free drug [7].

The oral bioavailability of Curcumin was improved by incorporation into solid lipid nanoparticles composed of soy lecithin, the nanoparticles were spherical with a high entrapment efficiency and good stability after storage for 12 months at 5 °C [8]. Also, solid lipid nanoparticles enhance the stability of curcuminoids [68].

Diosmin, an insoluble natural flavonoid, was nanoencapsulated, in combination with different essential oils Rosmarinus officinalis (Rosemary oil), Zingiber officinale (Ginger oil), and Vitis vinifera (Grapeseed oil). The lipid nanoparticles showed a promising anti-aging, anti-oxidant, and photoprotective effect [16].

Triptolide (TP) isolated from the *Tripterygium wilfordii* Hook. F (Celastraceae) was loaded in solid lipid nanoparticles and had the potential to penetrate into the skin and showed efficacy for the treatment of certain cases like inflammatory and autoimmune diseases [69].

Vesicular Nanoparticles

The vesicular structure consists of highly ordered assemblies with one or more concentric lipid bilayer composed of amphiphilic ingredients and water, it is able to incorporate both hydrophilic and hydrophobic compounds [70]. Vesicular nanosystems have many advantages like extended drug effects, toxicity reduction, targeted drug delivery, and enhancement of drug bioavailability [71].

Liposomes are spherical vesicles rich in cholesterol and phospholipids developed since 1970 for targeted drug delivery. This delivery system has enhanced the effect of many drugs of plant origin.

Silymarin widely used in the treatment of different liver diseases is obtained from the seeds of *Silybum marianum* (Compositae). It was formulated in hybrid liposomes composed of lecithin, cholesterol, stearylamine, and Tween 20 for buccal administration to overcome its low oral bioavailability. The liposomal silymarin showed a high hepato-protective effect against carbon tetrachloride-induced toxicity [72].

Quercetin-loaded liposomes were prepared using egg phosphatidylcholine, cholesterol for intranasal administration. The intranasal liposomes attained higher cognitive and anxiolytic effects compared to the drug suspension and orally administered liposomes, this was attributed to the higher alteration of various neurotransmitters [73].

Although liposomes are offering some advantages for drug delivery, they also have some disadvantages related to physicochemical instability (aggregation, sedimentation, fusion), problems of sterilization and large-scale production; therefore some other types of vesicular nanoparticles were developed [6]. Kamel *et al.* developed a proniosomal gel for the natural flavonoid rutin for rectal administration [74]. Proniosomes are niosomal hybrids, which upon hydration are transformed into niosomes. Proniosomes are composed of phospholipids and nonionic surfactants, which can act as penetration enhancers. Also, proniosomes have some advantages like ease of transportation and storage. They also avoid many problems associated with the niosomes (*i.e.*, aggregation), or the liposomes (degradation by hydrolysis or oxidation, sedimentation, aggregation) in addition to high production costs, problems concerning the purity of phospholipids, in addition to difficulty of large-scale production. In this study, different mixtures of Gelucire 50/13 or Gelucire 44/14 and Span 60 were used to prepare the proniosomal gel. The optimized preparation attained the suitable release profile and has the capability to accumulate within the rectal wall [74]. Different vesicular systems were investigated to improve the ocular therapeutic potential of the multi-function flavonoid Baicalin [75].

Phytosomes are lipidic complexes consisting of phosphatidylcholine together with the herbal component. Some studies reported the enhanced bioavailability of some herbal extracts like Ginseng, Curcumin, Green tea, Ginko Biloba, and quercetin by promoting the permeation of biological membranes [5].

NANOEMULSIONS

Nanoemulsions are homogenous and thermodynamically stable preparations with a transparent or translucent appearance. They are composed of oil, surfactant, co-surfactant, and water. They can incorporate lipophilic as well as hydrophilic drugs [76] and can protect the drug from oxidation, degradation, and hydrolysis. Also, extended drug release can be obtained [77].

Clove oil was prepared in the form of an o/w nanoemulsions and had good stability with a high anti-fungal effect compared to the crude clove oil [78]. In the same trend, other oils like neem and citronella oils-loaded nanoemulsions showed a good antifungal activity [79].

Kamel and Basha prepared a liquisolid self-emulsifying drug delivery system of Rutin which showed a significantly higher drug release compared to the drug suspension [80]. These systems consisted of different nanoemulsions loaded into solid nano-structured carriers (Neusilin®, Fujicalin®, and F-melt®).

MICELLAR NANOPARTICLES

Micellar nanosystems consist of amphiphilic block copolymers arranged to form a core-shell structure in aqueous solutions. Hydrophobic agents are placed in the hydrophobic core, while hydrophilic ones are incorporated in the hydrophilic shell and the whole system is soluble in an aqueous environment [81].

Curcumin was loaded into monomethoxy poly(ethylene glycol)-poly(ε-caprolactone) micelles and showed good angiogenesis inhibition [82].

In another recent study, Resveratrol was loaded in a co-micellar nanosystem and showed a significantly higher drug release and anti-arthritic effect compared to the drug suspension [33].

HYBRID NANOPARTICLES

Hybrid nanoparticles are mixed nanosystems offering combined advantages or even synergistic effects, in addition to the mitigation of the limitations associated with some nanostructured systems. Various methods of preparation are possible for the formation of this type of nanoparticles [83].

Lipophilic gold nanorods and curcumin were loaded into polymeric nanomicelles composed of biocompatible PLGA-PEG copolymer and showed to be effective in safe and effective in the treatment of premalignant esophageal adenocarcinoma [84].

Biocompatible halloysite nanotubes coated with bio-adhesive chitosan and loaded with curcumin showed an efficient anti-cancer activity and was suitable as a cell-targeted anti-cancer delivery platform [85].

Rutin/TiO_2 nano-cream was investigated as a sun-block, the combination of organic/inorganic active components attained a higher sun protection factor compared to Rutin nano-cream [7].

Resveratrol was loaded in a PLA-coated co-micellar system and showed a higher efficacy as site-specific anti-arthritic compared to the un-coated nanosystems based on the analysis of biochemical markers as well as histopathological studies [33].

CONCLUSION

Phytotherapeutics provide multiple benefits for healthcare. Their safety, availability, and low cost are distinguishable features. However, their complicated structure, difficult validation methods, unspecified dosage, and low aqueous solubility are great confrontations. Nanotechnology-based as well as some novel drug delivery systems have proven to be a worthy weapon to mitigate these limitations. However, much effort and huge investment into academic research are awaited to overcome barriers to nanotechnology-based systems industrial production, specifically, safety issues, scalability, and reproducibility.

There are no known conflicts of interest associated with this publication and there has been no significant financial support for this work that could have influenced its outcome.

CONFLICT OF INTEREST

The author declares that there is no conflict of interest in this chapter.

CONSENT FOR PUBLICATION

Not applicable.

ACKNOWLEDGEMENTS

Declared none.

REFERENCES

[1] Saklani A, Kutty SK. Plant-derived compounds in clinical trials. Drug Discov Today 2008; 13(3-4): 161-71.
[http://dx.doi.org/10.1016/j.drudis.2007.10.010] [PMID: 18275914]

[2] Bonifácio BV, Silva PB, Ramos MA, Negri KMS, Bauab TM, Chorilli M. Nanotechnology-based drug delivery systems and herbal medicines: a review. Int J Nanomedicine 2014; 9: 1-15.
[PMID: 24363556]

[3] Pundir S, Badola A, Sharma D. Sustained release matrix technology and recent advance in matrix drug delivery system: a review. International Journal of drug research and technology 2017; 3(1): 8.

[4] Kesarwani K, Gupta R, Mukerjee A. Bioavailability enhancers of herbal origin: an overview. Asian Pac J Trop Biomed 2013; 3(4): 253-66.
[http://dx.doi.org/10.1016/S2221-1691(13)60060-X] [PMID: 23620848]

[5] Ajazuddin , Saraf S. Applications of novel drug delivery system for herbal formulations. Fitoterapia 2010; 81(7): 680-9.
[http://dx.doi.org/10.1016/j.fitote.2010.05.001] [PMID: 20471457]

[6] Musthaba SM, Baboota S, Ahmed S, Ahuja A, Ali J. Status of novel drug delivery technology for phytotherapeutics. Expert Opin Drug Deliv 2009; 6(6): 625-37.
[http://dx.doi.org/10.1517/17425240902980154] [PMID: 19505192]

[7] Kamel R, Mostafa DM. Rutin nanostructured lipid cosmeceutical preparation with sun protective potential. J Photochem Photobiol B 2015; 153: 59-66.
[http://dx.doi.org/10.1016/j.jphotobiol.2015.09.002] [PMID: 26398812]

[8] Kakkar V, Singh S, Singla D, Kaur IP. Exploring solid lipid nanoparticles to enhance the oral bioavailability of curcumin. Mol Nutr Food Res 2011; 55(3): 495-503.
[http://dx.doi.org/10.1002/mnfr.201000310] [PMID: 20938993]

[9] Asfour MH, Mohsen AM. Formulation and evaluation of pH-sensitive rutin nanospheres against colon carcinoma using HCT-116 cell line. J Adv Res 2017; 9: 17-26.
[http://dx.doi.org/10.1016/j.jare.2017.10.003] [PMID: 30034879]

[10] Kamel R, Basha M. Preparation and *in vitro* evaluation of rutin nanostructured liquisolid delivery system. Bull Fac Pharm Cairo Univ 2013; 51(2): 261-72.
[http://dx.doi.org/10.1016/j.bfopcu.2013.08.002]

[11] Oliveira CA, Peres DDA, Graziola F, *et al.* Cutaneous biocompatible rutin-loaded gelatin-based nanoparticles increase the SPF of the association of UVA and UVB filters. Eur J Pharm Sci 2016; 81: 1-9.
[http://dx.doi.org/10.1016/j.ejps.2015.09.016] [PMID: 26428697]

[12] Ahmad N, Ahmad R, Naqvi AA, *et al.* Rutin-encapsulated chitosan nanoparticles targeted to the brain in the treatment of Cerebral Ischemia. Int J Biol Macromol 2016; 91: 640-55.
[http://dx.doi.org/10.1016/j.ijbiomac.2016.06.001] [PMID: 27264648]

[13] Ramaswamy S, Dwarampudi LP, Kadiyala M, *et al.* Formulation and characterization of chitosan encapsulated phytoconstituents of curcumin and rutin nanoparticles. Int J Biol Macromol 2017; 104(Pt B): 1807-12.
[http://dx.doi.org/10.1016/j.ijbiomac.2017.06.112] [PMID: 28668610]

[14] Patil AG, Jobanputra AH. Rutin-chitosan nanoparticles: fabrication, characterization and application in dental disorders. Polym Plast Technol Eng 2015; 54(2): 202-8.

[http://dx.doi.org/10.1080/03602559.2014.935425]

[15] Almeida JS, Lima F, Ros SD, Bulhões LO, de Carvalho LM, Beck RC. Nanostructured systems containing rutin: *in vitro* antioxidant activity and photostability studies. Nanoscale Res Lett 2010; 5(10): 1603-10.
[http://dx.doi.org/10.1007/s11671-010-9683-1] [PMID: 21076700]

[16] Kamel R, Abbas H, Fayez A. Diosmin/essential oil combination for dermal photo-protection using a lipoid colloidal carrier. J Photochem Photobiol B 2017; 170: 49-57.
[http://dx.doi.org/10.1016/j.jphotobiol.2017.03.019] [PMID: 28390258]

[17] Freag MS, Elnaggar YS, Abdallah OY. Development of novel polymer-stabilized diosmin nanosuspensions: *in vitro* appraisal and *ex vivo* permeation. Int J Pharm 2013; 454(1): 462-71.
[http://dx.doi.org/10.1016/j.ijpharm.2013.06.039] [PMID: 23830765]

[18] El Hady WEA, Mohamed EA, Soliman OAE-A. Int J Nanomedicine 2019; 14: 7191.
[http://dx.doi.org/10.2147/IJN.S213836] [PMID: 31564873]

[19] Atia NM, Hazzah HA, Gaafar PME, Abdallah OY. Diosmin Nanocrystal-Loaded Wafers for Treatment of Diabetic Ulcer: *In Vitro* and *In Vivo* Evaluation. J Pharm Sci 2019; 108(5): 1857-71.
[http://dx.doi.org/10.1016/j.xphs.2018.12.019] [PMID: 30599171]

[20] Montenegro L, Paolino D, Drago R, Pignatello R, Fresta M, Puglisi G. Influence of liposome composition on *in vitro* permeation of diosmin through human stratum corneum and epidermis. J Drug Deliv Sci Technol 2006; 16(2): 133-40.
[http://dx.doi.org/10.1016/S1773-2247(06)50020-6]

[21] Cheng KK, Yeung CF, Ho SW, Chow SF, Chow AH, Baum L. Highly stabilized curcumin nanoparticles tested in an *in vitro* blood-brain barrier model and in Alzheimer's disease Tg2576 mice. AAPS J 2013; 15(2): 324-36.
[http://dx.doi.org/10.1208/s12248-012-9444-4] [PMID: 23229335]

[22] Duan J, Zhang Y, Han S, *et al.* Synthesis and *in vitro/in vivo* anti-cancer evaluation of curcumin-loaded chitosan/poly(butyl cyanoacrylate) nanoparticles. Int J Pharm 2010; 400(1-2): 211-20.
[http://dx.doi.org/10.1016/j.ijpharm.2010.08.033] [PMID: 20813175]

[23] Deljoo S, Rabiee N, Rabiee M. Curcumin-hybrid nanoparticles in drug delivery system. Asian Journal of Nanosciences and Materials 2019; 2(1, pp. 1-119): 66-91.

[24] Kim TH, Jiang HH, Youn YS, *et al.* Preparation and characterization of water-soluble albumin-bound curcumin nanoparticles with improved antitumor activity. Int J Pharm 2011; 403(1-2): 285-91.
[http://dx.doi.org/10.1016/j.ijpharm.2010.10.041] [PMID: 21035530]

[25] Yallapu MM, Maher DM, Sundram V, Bell MC, Jaggi M, Chauhan SC. Curcumin induces chemo/radio-sensitization in ovarian cancer cells and curcumin nanoparticles inhibit ovarian cancer cell growth. J Ovarian Res 2010; 3(1): 11.
[http://dx.doi.org/10.1186/1757-2215-3-11] [PMID: 20429876]

[26] Zhao Z, Xie M, Li Y, *et al.* Formation of curcumin nanoparticles *via* solution-enhanced dispersion by supercritical CO_2. Int J Nanomedicine 2015; 10: 3171-81.
[http://dx.doi.org/10.2147/IJN.S80434] [PMID: 25995627]

[27] Pandita D, Kumar S, Poonia N, Lather V. Solid lipid nanoparticles enhance oral bioavailability of resveratrol, a natural polyphenol. Food Res Int 2014; 62: 1165-74.
[http://dx.doi.org/10.1016/j.foodres.2014.05.059]

[28] Gokce EH, Korkmaz E, Dellera E, Sandri G, Bonferoni MC, Ozer O. Resveratrol-loaded solid lipid nanoparticles versus nanostructured lipid carriers: evaluation of antioxidant potential for dermal applications. Int J Nanomedicine 2012; 7: 1841-50.
[http://dx.doi.org/10.2147/IJN.S29710] [PMID: 22605933]

[29] Huang X, Dai Y, Cai J, Zhong N, Xiao H, McClements DJ, *et al.* Resveratrol encapsulation in core-shell biopolymer nanoparticles: Impact on antioxidant and anticancer activities. Food Hydrocoll 2017;

64: 157-65.
[http://dx.doi.org/10.1016/j.foodhyd.2016.10.029]

[30] Karthikeyan S, Prasad NR, Ganamani A, Balamurugan E. Anticancer activity of resveratrol-loaded gelatin nanoparticles on NCI-H460 non-small cell lung cancer cells. Biomedicine & Preventive Nutrition 2013; 3(1): 64-73.
[http://dx.doi.org/10.1016/j.bionut.2012.10.009]

[31] Abbas H, Kamel R. Potential role of resveratrol-loaded elastic sorbitan monostearate nanovesicles for the prevention of UV-induced skin damage. J Liposome Res 2019; 1-9.
[PMID: 30741053]

[32] Abbas H, Kamel R, El-Sayed N. Dermal anti-oxidant, anti-inflammatory and anti-aging effects of Compritol ATO-based Resveratrol colloidal carriers prepared using mixed surfactants. Int J Pharm 2018; 541(1-2): 37-47.
[http://dx.doi.org/10.1016/j.ijpharm.2018.01.054] [PMID: 29458209]

[33] Kamel R, Abbas H, Shaffie NM. Development and evaluation of PLA-coated co-micellar nanosystem of Resveratrol for the intra-articular treatment of arthritis. Int J Pharm 2019; 569118560
[http://dx.doi.org/10.1016/j.ijpharm.2019.118560] [PMID: 31351180]

[34] Sokolsky-Papkov M, Agashi K, Olaye A, Shakesheff K, Domb AJ. Polymer carriers for drug delivery in tissue engineering. Adv Drug Deliv Rev 2007; 59(4-5): 187-206.
[http://dx.doi.org/10.1016/j.addr.2007.04.001] [PMID: 17540473]

[35] Xiaoyan A, Jun Y, Min W, *et al.* Preparation of chitosan-gelatin scaffold containing tetrandrine-loaded nano-aggregates and its controlled release behavior. Int J Pharm 2008; 350(1-2): 257-64.
[http://dx.doi.org/10.1016/j.ijpharm.2007.09.008] [PMID: 17945449]

[36] Jouybar A, Seyedjafari E, Ardeshirylajimi A, *et al.* Enhanced skin regeneration by herbal extract-coated poly-L-lactic acid nanofibrous scaffold. Artif Organs 2017; 41(11): E296-307.
[http://dx.doi.org/10.1111/aor.12926] [PMID: 28621889]

[37] Khakestani M, Jafari SH, Zahedi P, Bagheri R, Hajiaghaee R. Physical, morphological, and biological studies on PLA/n HA composite nanofibrous webs containing E quisetum arvense herbal extract for bone tissue engineering. J Appl Polym Sci 2017; 134(39): 45343.
[http://dx.doi.org/10.1002/app.45343]

[38] Annapoorna M, Sudheesh Kumar PT, Lakshman LR, Lakshmanan V-K, Nair SV, Jayakumar R. Biochemical properties of Hemigraphis alternata incorporated chitosan hydrogel scaffold. Carbohydr Polym 2013; 92(2): 1561-5.
[http://dx.doi.org/10.1016/j.carbpol.2012.10.041] [PMID: 23399189]

[39] Soumya S, Sajesh K, Jayakumar R, Nair S, Chennazhi K. Development of a phytochemical scaffold for bone tissue engineering using Cissus quadrangularis extract. Carbohydr Polym 2012; 87(2): 1787-95.
[http://dx.doi.org/10.1016/j.carbpol.2011.09.094]

[40] Cai K, Yao K, Yang Z, Li X. Surface modification of three-dimensional poly(d,l-lactic acid) scaffolds with baicalin: a histological study. Acta Biomater 2007; 3(4): 597-605.
[http://dx.doi.org/10.1016/j.actbio.2006.12.005] [PMID: 17291842]

[41] Suganya S, Senthil Ram T, Lakshmi B, Giridev V. Herbal drug incorporated antibacterial nanofibrous mat fabricated by electrospinning: an excellent matrix for wound dressings. J Appl Polym Sci 2011; 121(5): 2893-9.
[http://dx.doi.org/10.1002/app.33915]

[42] Suganya S, Venugopal J, Ramakrishna S, Lakshmi B, Giri Dev V. Herbally derived polymeric nanofibrous scaffolds for bone tissue regeneration. J Appl Polym Sci 2014; 131(3)
[http://dx.doi.org/10.1002/app.39835]

[43] Biswas A, Amarajeewa M, Senapati S, Sahu M, Maiti P. Sustained release of herbal drugs using

biodegradable scaffold for faster wound healing and better patient compliance. Nanomedicine (Lond) 2018; 14(7): 2131-41.
[http://dx.doi.org/10.1016/j.nano.2018.07.003] [PMID: 30031095]

[44] Chen Y, Lin X, Park H, Greever R. Study of artemisinin nanocapsules as anticancer drug delivery systems. Nanomedicine (Lond) 2009; 5(3): 316-22.
[http://dx.doi.org/10.1016/j.nano.2008.12.005] [PMID: 19523432]

[45] Brigger I, Dubernet C, Couvreur P. Nanoparticles in cancer therapy and diagnosis. Adv Drug Deliv Rev 2012; 64: 24-36.
[http://dx.doi.org/10.1016/j.addr.2012.09.006] [PMID: 12204596]

[46] Mainardes RM, Gremião MPD, Evangelista RC. Thermoanalytical study of praziquantel-loaded PLGA nanoparticles. Revista Brasileira de Ciências Farmacêuticas 2006; 42(4): 523-30.
[http://dx.doi.org/10.1590/S1516-93322006000400007]

[47] Kamel R. Nanotherapeutics as promising approaches to combat fungal infections. Drug Development Research
[http://dx.doi.org/10.1002/ddr.21533]

[48] Liu M, Dong J, Yang Y, Yang X, Xu H. Anti-inflammatory effects of triptolide loaded poly(D,L-lactic acid) nanoparticles on adjuvant-induced arthritis in rats. J Ethnopharmacol 2005; 97(2): 219-25.
[http://dx.doi.org/10.1016/j.jep.2004.10.031] [PMID: 15707756]

[49] Min KH, Park K, Kim Y-S, *et al.* Hydrophobically modified glycol chitosan nanoparticles-encapsulated camptothecin enhance the drug stability and tumor targeting in cancer therapy. J Control Release 2008; 127(3): 208-18.
[http://dx.doi.org/10.1016/j.jconrel.2008.01.013] [PMID: 18336946]

[50] Zeisser-Labouèbe M, Lange N, Gurny R, Delie F. Hypericin-loaded nanoparticles for the photodynamic treatment of ovarian cancer. Int J Pharm 2006; 326(1-2): 174-81.
[http://dx.doi.org/10.1016/j.ijpharm.2006.07.012] [PMID: 16930882]

[51] Zhang L, Kosaraju SL. Biopolymeric delivery system for controlled release of polyphenolic antioxidants. Eur Polym J 2007; 43(7): 2956-66.
[http://dx.doi.org/10.1016/j.eurpolymj.2007.04.033]

[52] Bhatia A, Shard P, Chopra D, Mishra T. Chitosan nanoparticles as Carrier of Immunorestoratory plant extract: synthesis, characterization and Immunorestoratory efficacy. Int J Drug Deliv 2011; 3(2): 381-5.

[53] Yen F-L, Wu T-H, Lin L-T, Cham T-M, Lin C-C. Nanoparticles formulation of Cuscuta chinensis prevents acetaminophen-induced hepatotoxicity in rats. Food Chem Toxicol 2008; 46(5): 1771-7.
[http://dx.doi.org/10.1016/j.fct.2008.01.021] [PMID: 18308443]

[54] Rajendran R, Radhai R, Kotresh TM, Csiszar E. Development of antimicrobial cotton fabrics using herb loaded nanoparticles. Carbohydr Polym 2013; 91(2): 613-7.
[http://dx.doi.org/10.1016/j.carbpol.2012.08.064] [PMID: 23121954]

[55] Kamel R, Salama A, Shaffie N, Salah N. Cerebral effect of optimized *Allium sativum* oil-loaded chitosan nanorods: GC-MS analysis and *in-vitro/in-vivo* evaluation. Food and Function 2020.

[56] Bisht S, Feldmann G, Soni S, *et al.* Polymeric nanoparticle-encapsulated curcumin ("nanocurcumin"): a novel strategy for human cancer therapy. J Nanobiotechnology 2007; 5(1): 3.
[http://dx.doi.org/10.1186/1477-3155-5-3] [PMID: 17439648]

[57] Mukerjee A, Vishwanatha JK. Formulation, characterization and evaluation of curcumin-loaded PLGA nanospheres for cancer therapy. Anticancer Res 2009; 29(10): 3867-75.
[PMID: 19846921]

[58] Bhawana , Basniwal RK, Buttar HS, Jain VK, Jain N. Curcumin nanoparticles: preparation, characterization, and antimicrobial study. J Agric Food Chem 2011; 59(5): 2056-61.
[http://dx.doi.org/10.1021/jf104402t] [PMID: 21322563]

[59] Zheng X, Kan B, Gou M, *et al.* Preparation of MPEG-PLA nanoparticle for honokiol delivery *in vitro*. Int J Pharm 2010; 386(1-2): 262-7.
[http://dx.doi.org/10.1016/j.ijpharm.2009.11.014] [PMID: 19932160]

[60] Khuda-Bukhsh AR, Bhattacharyya SS, Paul S, Boujedaini N. Polymeric nanoparticle encapsulation of a naturally occurring plant scopoletin and its effects on human melanoma cell A375. J Chin Integr Med 2010; 8(9): 853-62.
[http://dx.doi.org/10.3736/jcim20100909] [PMID: 20836976]

[61] Moulari B, Lboutounne H, Chaumont J-P, Guillaume Y, Millet J, Pellequer Y. Potentiation of the bactericidal activity of Harungana madagascariensis Lam. ex Poir. (Hypericaceae) leaf extract against oral bacteria using poly (D, L-lactide-co-glycolide) nanoparticles: *in vitro* study. Acta Odontol Scand 2006; 64(3): 153-8.
[http://dx.doi.org/10.1080/00016350500483152] [PMID: 16809192]

[62] Wu T-H, Yen F-L, Lin L-T, Tsai T-R, Lin C-C, Cham T-M. Preparation, physicochemical characterization, and antioxidant effects of quercetin nanoparticles. Int J Pharm 2008; 346(1-2): 160-8.
[http://dx.doi.org/10.1016/j.ijpharm.2007.06.036] [PMID: 17689897]

[63] Pardeike J, Hommoss A, Müller RH. Lipid nanoparticles (SLN, NLC) in cosmetic and pharmaceutical dermal products. Int J Pharm 2009; 366(1-2): 170-84.
[http://dx.doi.org/10.1016/j.ijpharm.2008.10.003] [PMID: 18992314]

[64] Müller RH, Radtke M, Wissing SA. Solid lipid nanoparticles (SLN) and nanostructured lipid carriers (NLC) in cosmetic and dermatological preparations. Adv Drug Deliv Rev 2002; 54 (Suppl. 1): S131-55.
[http://dx.doi.org/10.1016/S0169-409X(02)00118-7] [PMID: 12460720]

[65] Mehnert W, Mäder K. Solid lipid nanoparticles: production, characterization and applications. Adv Drug Deliv Rev 2012; 64: 83-101.
[http://dx.doi.org/10.1016/j.addr.2012.09.021] [PMID: 11311991]

[66] Li H, Zhao X, Ma Y, Zhai G, Li L, Lou H. Enhancement of gastrointestinal absorption of quercetin by solid lipid nanoparticles. J Control Release 2009; 133(3): 238-44.
[http://dx.doi.org/10.1016/j.jconrel.2008.10.002] [PMID: 18951932]

[67] Chen-yu G, Chun-fen Y, Qi-lu L, *et al.* Development of a quercetin-loaded nanostructured lipid carrier formulation for topical delivery. Int J Pharm 2012; 430(1-2): 292-8.
[http://dx.doi.org/10.1016/j.ijpharm.2012.03.042] [PMID: 22486962]

[68] Tiyaboonchai W, Tungpradit W, Plianbangchang P. Formulation and characterization of curcuminoids loaded solid lipid nanoparticles. Int J Pharm 2007; 337(1-2): 299-306.
[http://dx.doi.org/10.1016/j.ijpharm.2006.12.043] [PMID: 17287099]

[69] Mei Z, Chen H, Weng T, Yang Y, Yang X. Solid lipid nanoparticle and microemulsion for topical delivery of triptolide. Eur J Pharm Biopharm 2003; 56(2): 189-96.
[http://dx.doi.org/10.1016/S0939-6411(03)00067-5] [PMID: 12957632]

[70] in. British Pharmacopoeia. London 1993; pp. 159-60.

[71] Jadhav SM, Morey P, Karpe M, Kadam V. Novel vesicular system: an overview. J Appl Pharm Sci 2012; 2(01): 193-202.

[72] El-Samaligy MS, Afifi NN, Mahmoud EA. Increasing bioavailability of silymarin using a buccal liposomal delivery system: preparation and experimental design investigation. Int J Pharm 2006; 308(1-2): 140-8.
[http://dx.doi.org/10.1016/j.ijpharm.2005.11.006] [PMID: 16356669]

[73] Priprem A, Watanatorn J, Sutthiparinyanont S, Phachonpai W, Muchimapura S. Anxiety and cognitive effects of quercetin liposomes in rats. Nanomedicine (Lond) 2008; 4(1): 70-8.
[http://dx.doi.org/10.1016/j.nano.2007.12.001] [PMID: 18249157]

[74] Kamel R, Basha M, Abd El-Alim SH. Development of a novel vesicular system using a binary mixture of sorbitan monostearate and polyethylene glycol fatty acid esters for rectal delivery of rutin. J Liposome Res 2013; 23(1): 28-36.
[http://dx.doi.org/10.3109/08982104.2012.727422] [PMID: 23083098]

[75] Ashraf O, Nasr M, Nebsen M, Said AMA, Sammour O. *In vitro* stabilization and *in vivo* improvement of ocular pharmacokinetics of the multi-therapeutic agent baicalin: Delineating the most suitable vesicular systems. Int J Pharm 2018; 539(1-2): 83-94.
[http://dx.doi.org/10.1016/j.ijpharm.2018.01.041] [PMID: 29374518]

[76] Lee PJ, Langer R, Shastri VP. Novel microemulsion enhancer formulation for simultaneous transdermal delivery of hydrophilic and hydrophobic drugs. Pharm Res 2003; 20(2): 264-9.
[http://dx.doi.org/10.1023/A:1022283423116] [PMID: 12636166]

[77] Kogan A, Garti N. Microemulsions as transdermal drug delivery vehicles. Adv Colloid Interface Sci 2006; 123-126: 369-85.
[http://dx.doi.org/10.1016/j.cis.2006.05.014] [PMID: 16843424]

[78] Wan J, Zhong S, Schwarz P, Chen B, Rao J. Influence of oil phase composition on the antifungal and mycotoxin inhibitory activity of clove oil nanoemulsions. Food Funct 2018; 9(5): 2872-82.
[http://dx.doi.org/10.1039/C7FO02073B] [PMID: 29713695]

[79] Ali EOM, Shakil NA, Rana VS, Sarkar DJ, Majumder S, Kaushik P, *et al.* Antifungal activity of nano emulsions of neem and citronella oils against phytopathogenic fungi, Rhizoctonia solani and Sclerotium rolfsii. Ind Crops Prod 2017; 108: 379-87.
[http://dx.doi.org/10.1016/j.indcrop.2017.06.061]

[80] Kamel R, Basha M. Preparation and *in vitro* evaluation of rutin nanostructured liquisolid delivery system. Bulletin of Faculty of Pharmacy 2013; 51: 261-72.
[http://dx.doi.org/10.1016/j.bfopcu.2013.08.002]

[81] Wakaskar RR. Polymeric micelles for drug delivery. Int J Drug Dev Res 2017; 9: 01-2.

[82] Gou M, Men K, Shi H, *et al.* Curcumin-loaded biodegradable polymeric micelles for colon cancer therapy *in vitro* and *in vivo*. Nanoscale 2011; 3(4): 1558-67.
[http://dx.doi.org/10.1039/c0nr00758g] [PMID: 21283869]

[83] Mandal B, Bhattacharjee H, Mittal N, *et al.* Core-shell-type lipid-polymer hybrid nanoparticles as a drug delivery platform. Nanomedicine (Lond) 2013; 9(4): 474-91.
[http://dx.doi.org/10.1016/j.nano.2012.11.010] [PMID: 23261500]

[84] Martin RC, Locatelli E, Li Y, *et al.* Gold nanorods and curcumin-loaded nanomicelles for efficient *in vivo* photothermal therapy of Barrett's esophagus. Nanomedicine (Lond) 2015; 10(11): 1723-33.
[http://dx.doi.org/10.2217/nnm.15.25] [PMID: 25706349]

[85] Rao KM, Kumar A, Suneetha M, Han SS. pH and near-infrared active; chitosan-coated halloysite nanotubes loaded with curcumin-Au hybrid nanoparticles for cancer drug delivery. Int J Biol Macromol 2018; 112: 119-25.
[http://dx.doi.org/10.1016/j.ijbiomac.2018.01.163] [PMID: 29378273]

SUBJECT INDEX

A

D

E

F

M

N

O

S

T

U

V

W

Y

Z

Made in the USA
Las Vegas, NV
03 November 2026

57422838R00109